PATHWAYS TO WELLNESS

FOR THE LOVE OF
LIVING

A Fresh Approach to
Nutrition, Weight Loss, & Exercise

JANICE MAST

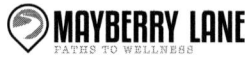

Copyright © 2016 Mayberry Lane

All rights reserved. This book or any portion thereof may not be reproduced or used in any manner whatsoever without the express written permission of the publisher except for the use of brief quotations in a book review.

First Printing, 2016

ISBN: 978-1-946389-00-8

Printed in the United States of America

May this book be a tool

to guide you and your

loved ones towards the

path to wellness.

This information is presented solely for educational purposes.

Consult your doctor if you have any pre-existing conditions before starting a diet or exercise routine.

CONTENTS

PART I - **NUTRITION**

Chapter 1
INTRODUCTION TO NUTRITION 13

Chapter 2
THE 4 PILLARS 21

Chapter 3
THE SCIENCE OF FOOD 31
    Nutrition Basics *31*
    Carbs *41*
    Fat *48*
    Protein *52*
    Vitamins, Minerals & Phytochemicals *57*
    Liquids *61*

Chapter 4
MAKING IT WORK 67
    Meal Planning *67*
    Should I Buy Organic? *68*
    Incorporating More Fruits & Vegetables *71*
    How to Build Flavor Naturally *73*
    Smarter Snacking *75*

RECIPES 77
RECIPE INDEX 114

PART II - **EXERCISE**

Chapter 5
INTRODUCTION TO EXERCISE 119

Chapter 6
LEARNING ABOUT EXERCISE 123
    The Benefits & Importance of Exercise 123
    How Much Exercise Do I Need for My Age & Condition? 130
    Activities and Levels of Exertion 135
    Exercise and Nutrition 141

Chapter 7
GETTING STARTED 147

Chapter 8
GETTING ACTIVE 157
    Everyday Exercise for the Whole Family 157
    Stretching 160
    Strength Training for All Levels 163
    Running 181
    Other Exercises You Can Do At Home 186

Chapter 9
EXERCISING TO LOSE WEIGHT 191

Chapter 10
TRACKING YOUR PROGRESS 197

FREQUENTLY ASKED QUESTIONS 199
STATISTICS & FACTS 205

PART III - **WEIGHT LOSS**

Chapter 11
INTRODUCTION TO WEIGHT LOSS 213

Chapter 12
SET A GOAL 221

Chapter 13
THE PLAN 225
    Choose Your Phase *225*
    Tips *226*
    Meal Plan Guidelines *229*
    Meal Plans *231*
    Substitutes *234*
    Snack Options *235*
    Exercise Plans *236*

FREQUENTLY ASKED QUESTIONS 243
SOURCES 250

PART ONE
NUTRITION

Chapter One
INTRODUCTION TO NUTRITION

Does health feel like a popular fad right now? Does it overwhelm you to try and decide which method to follow - vegan, organic, gluten-free, or Paleo? For those of you who would like to lose weight, there are a wide variety of other options to choose from such as the Atkins, Weight Watchers, grapefruit, or no-salt diets. There are so many options out there; it can seem that as soon as you begin making changes, new things are being recommended.

Every few years there is a new food bad guy that researchers say you should avoid. In the 1970s, no one questioned whether eggs were the heart-attack risk about which nutritionists warned us. Now, of course, eggs have become such a cherished food that many people raise their own laying hens. Such examples of food confusion and misinformation abound.

There was a time when whole, healthy foods were the norm and were also very accessible. The problem we in the Western world have encountered is that we have allowed food companies, advertisers, and food researchers to do our thinking for us. Sadly, food production thrives more on the interest in profit than in concern for our well-being.

So how do we get back to a wholesome way of eating? This guide helps break down the walls of myth and confusion that surround healthy living, and gives you simple steps to incorporate healthy nutrition into your family's life. This is not done with another temporary diet, but as a new lifestyle that you can stick with for the future. This approach is based on eating a variety of nutritious foods in a well-balanced diet. It does not restrict certain food groups or ban sweets. Healthy eating is not meant to be a complicated or restrictive diet but rather, it follows a few basic guidelines that will nourish and fuel your body.

There are so many things that your bodies are meant to do; work, care for and play with your children, climb mountains, live long lives, and accomplish great things. Everyone deserves to have the optimum health that allows them to follow their dreams.

You may be afraid that this new lifestyle might require that you eat salad for the rest of your life and never enjoy a donut again. That is what keeps most people from eating healthier; the refusal to deprive themselves of enjoying their food. However, when you cleanse your system of the foods that make you feel heavy and over-stimulated, you will be able to notice the difference in how much better you feel when you eat fresh foods. With our extensive, locally tested and approved whole-food recipes we guarantee that you will not go hungry and that your taste buds will be happy. Choosing a new, healthy lifestyle also means that there is still a time and place for baked goods and desserts. The key to living healthy is educating yourself on the quality of your foods and how they nourish your body, in order to make better choices.

Introduction to Nutrition

Are you ready to get started? This is the beginning of a lifestyle change that will positively affect you and your family's life for the better. There's no reason to wait; let's dive into the world of delicious foods that we are meant to enjoy!

WHY BOTHER?

Nature's Design

Optimum Health

Increased Energy

Prevention of Disease

Weight Loss *(that stay's off)*

With each new diet plan comes an extensive theory on why it is the healthiest way of eating well and losing weight. People buy into these plans and theories with an investment of $40 billion a year in America. One would think this investment should provide a strategy that works, but it seems they just come, run their course, and then go out of style.

The reason why fad diets don't last long-term is that they typically involve cutting out a major food group that most people enjoy, are extensively restrictive, or involve a lot of calorie counting and meal planning. It's hard to restrict yourself from things that you love, and plans that take up too much time are hard to maintain. Even if some people can lose weight on these diets, they typically regain it after suspending the practice. Why? Because your body needs a diet that it can sustain over a lifetime, one that is wholesome and fulfilling to both to your body and your senses.

Eating wholesome should be simple – it is, in fact, how God created us to eat.

Fad diets may come and go, but a wholesome, well-rounded plan focused on whole foods is the key to optimal health, low disease risk, healthy weight, and long life. This approach provides the information you need to educate yourself about food and assists you in choosing a lifestyle of healthy eating. **Harvard refers to it as the "new nutrition," a way of eating that has been a matter of growing consensus over the last several decades, thanks to a hard-earned body of evidence.**

Researchers at Harvard are among those who have helped to establish that solid base of knowledge, which shows, among other things, just how powerful the effects of a healthful diet can be. Dr. Walter Willett, chair of the Department of Nutrition at Harvard T. H. Chang School of Public Health, one of the leading nutrition experts in the world, has devoted much of his career to understanding which aspects of diet play a role in optimal health. Willett says that diet not only plays a role in deterring heart disease and cancer, but also in the prevention of disease and dysfunction of almost every organ in the body including cataracts, infertility, and neurodegenerative (affecting nervous tissue) conditions.

This is encouraging news, seeing that you can prevent disease naturally through your diet instead of working backward with medications and treatments.

If you're convinced, there is no better time than now to start improving your health and well-being.

A LIFESTYLE OF NUTRITIOUS EATING

Many people are leery about changing their eating habits long-term because they think that they can no longer have the foods they enjoy. This is a legitimate concern. After all, why live a long life if you can't enjoy it? Often you will find that your cravings change when you eat nutritiously and your body is balanced – however, the key to maintaining this lifestyle is to allow yourself some of what you crave from time to time. We recommend following the 80/20 rule.

The reason why fad diets don't work is that their restrictive nature leaves you unsatisfied and hungry, which makes it hard to maintain. Another reason is that when you go on a restrictive diet and then return to unhealthy eating, you will easily and quickly regain the weight and often, even more. Eating healthy as a lifestyle will guarantee you the ability to maintain a healthy weight and still enjoy the foods you like.

We encourage you to give nutritious eating a chance and to challenge yourself to try new things. Our goal is to make understanding nutrition easy and getting started, simple. We have provided easy-to-follow guides for creating your own nutritious meals as well as a variety of meal plans with recipes for different taste preferences. With this guide, it has never been easier to wrap your head around the simplicity of nutrition and change your lifestyle for the better.

> # 80/20 RULE
>
> *Eat nutritiously 80% of the time.*
>
> *Allow yourself to eat your favorite*
>
> *less-nutritious foods 20% of the time.*

THE 80/20 RULE

This rule creates the balance that is so important to maintaining a lifestyle of nutritious eating. As we talk about in the whole foods section *(page 23)*, it is not toxic to eat less nutritious foods in your diet unless you make it the majority of what you eat.

This is **not** about becoming a *"health nut"* or jumping in the next *"fad diet"*. This **is** learning about food in order to make your own informed choices that fit you and your family longterm.

THE BASICS OF WHAT OUR BODIES NEED

The calories you consume in a day should be equal to or slightly less (500 calories) than the calories you burn, at which point you will lose weight. **You can stop here if you like.** *However,* what if you knew that your body needs certain nutrients, and poor food choices can affect your everyday and long-term health and energy? Less nutritious foods make it harder to eat less because you feel full for a shorter period of time, but eating the right foods along with calorie observation and exercise can multiply your weight loss.

It's important for you to know that eating "empty calories" – those sweet and delicious foods you crave - is not completely wrong. Thinking that it is wrong will lead you to become afraid of certain foods, form an unhealthy mindset, or cause you to feel overwhelmed at the thought of removing these foods permanently from your diet. Developing a new eating lifestyle doesn't mean that you can't ever have white sugar or flour. It doesn't mean that you have to ban red meat and butter. It just means that everyone can benefit from understanding the effects they have on our short and long-term health, and that making lifestyle changes can be easy and satisfying. Education and new habits are the keys here. This guide can be applied to every lifestyle, taste palette, and habit, and can help every individual find a style of eating that suits him or her. We believe that a nutritious lifestyle can be filling, delicious and rewarding.

NUTRITIOUS FOODS + EXERCISE

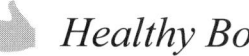 *Healthy Bodies*

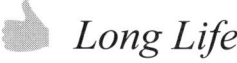 *Long Life*

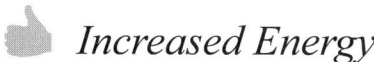 *Increased Energy*

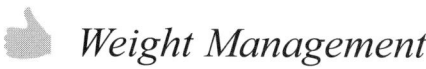 *Weight Management*

For the Love of Living

Chapter Two

THE 4 PILLARS
OF A NUTRITIOUS DIET

Remember these simple steps as a guide to changing your health for good.

STEP 1: EAT HEALTHY PROPORTIONS

Harvard University released a new eating chart in November of 2011 that moves meat away from the center of the plate and makes fruits and vegetables exactly half of what you eat.

To illustrate what a healthy diet should look like, nutrition experts at Harvard developed Harvard's Healthy Eating Plate. This diagram gives you basic guidance on food choices and shows you how to apportion foods on your plate. They state that, although every meal may not look like this plate - you may not have vegetables at breakfast, for instance - your meals over the course of the day should match these proportions.

FOLLOW THESE GUIDELINES: *(see chart on page 23)*

FRUITS & VEGETABLES - Half Plate
Fully half of the plate should contain fruits and vegetables. Most Americans don't get enough vegetables - the more you can add, the better. While you're at it, aim for a variety of colors and types. *(Note that for these purposes, potatoes – including French fries - don't count as vegetables.)*

WHOLE GRAINS - Quarter Plate
A quarter of the plate should be filled mostly with whole grains, limiting refined grains. Whole and intact grains, such as barley, quinoa, oats, and brown rice are better choices. Try to have at least half of your grains be whole grains.

HEALTHFUL PROTEIN - Quarter Plate
The final quarter of the plate should consist of healthful sources of protein, like fish, beans, nuts, seed, poultry, and eggs. High - fat meats and processed or cured meats don't appear here. Red meat and cheese should be limited.

HEALTHY OILS
The bottle on the left side is a reminder to use healthy oils like olive and canola in cooking, on salads, and at the table. Limit butter and saturated fats and avoid unhealthy trans fat (a mostly manufactured fat that is linked to an increased risk of heart disease).

WATER
The glass on the right side is a reminder to drink low - or no - calorie liquids like water, coffee, and tea. Skip sugary drinks and limit milk to one or two servings per day.

STAY ACTIVE
At the bottom is a reminder to stay active for good health and weight control.

The 4 Pillars

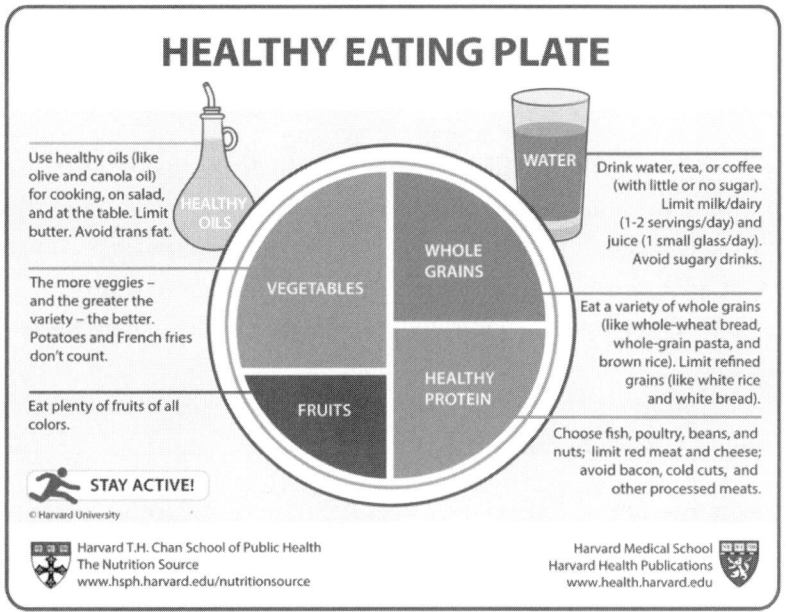

STEP 2: BASE DIET ON WHOLE FOODS

What are WHOLE foods?

Whole Foods: Foods that are closest to their naturally grown form, not processed or altered, or only minimally processed.[1]

Whole foods are usually 1-ingredient foods – like apples, oranges, blueberries, celery, peppers, almonds, nuts, and whole grains.

In this unprocessed form, fruits, vegetables, legumes, nuts, and whole grains contain a wealth of vital nutrients, such as fiber, vitamins, minerals, and phytochemicals (compounds with antioxidant and anti-inflammatory effects).

What are PROCESSED foods?

Processed Foods: Foods that are refined, stripped of many nutrients, and mixed with other ingredients to form new products.[1]

Processed foods are typically, but not always, those that are packaged, canned, boxed, and found at drive-throughs – like cereals, commercial orange juice, and American cheese.

Not all processing is bad. The kind of processing that we need to be aware of is that which reduces the vitamins, minerals, fiber, and phytochemicals in our food. According to Harvard, even healthful foods such as spinach, whole wheat, and beets become less nourishing when they are so heavily processed that they hardly resemble their original form. Some examples are the spinach in vegetable chips, the wheat in wheat bagels made from refined flour, and the beet sugar used in candy bars.

It is important to realize that processed foods are not necessarily always toxic, and a certain percentage can certainly be part of a healthy diet. However, if we are not taking in the nourishment that nature intended our bodies to receive, there will be negative consequences. A diet high in processed foods such as refined sugars and flour can cause blood sugar spikes resulting in low energy and an imbalance in our bodies systems. The thyroid, adrenal glands, reproductive glands, and digestive system are all susceptible to disruption by the consumption of unhealthy foods. High blood sugar is dangerously common among Americans and is the leading cause of type 2 diabetes. Another benefit of whole foods is that, in their whole form, they have the power to help protect your eyes, heart, brain, and more. When they are peeled, ground up, juiced, and stripped of various components - as they are in many processed foods - they lose a great deal of those valuable nutrients along the way. The peel and seeds are frequently discarded, and these, along with the fibrous pulp, are often the most highly concentrated sources of nutrients in the entire plant.

With processed foods, you end up with a serving of high-calorie foods with few nutrients in return. This is why it's so important to focus on nutrient-rich, whole foods.

STEP 3: **FOCUS ON PLANTS**

Although Harvard Health encourages Americans to remove meat from the center of their plate, recognize that you don't have to remove it all together. In their Healthy Eating Plate, however, plants take a much larger priority.

Why are plant foods so beneficial for your health? To begin with, they are rich in fiber, vitamins, minerals, healthy fats, and phytochemicals. Moreover, when you eat more of these plant foods, they tend to replace less healthful foods in your diet, such as fatty meats and high-fat dairy.

A plant-based diet can be as tasty as it is healthy. We know that if you've never eaten this way, it can be challenging to make this your habit, so Harvard Health gives some tips on how to make this easier.

- Turn your favorite meals into plant-based dishes. If you like lasagna, try eliminating the meat and substituting mushrooms and spinach. Use pinto beans instead of ground beef in your burritos.

- Find easy recipes for a few meatless dishes and aim to have them once or twice a week. Some ideas are vegetarian chili and veggie burgers.

- Instead of animal protein, eat at least 3 cups of legumes such as beans, lentils, and chickpeas every week. There are many ways to enjoy legumes. Toss chickpeas into a salad, add beans to a stew, or include lentils in a meatloaf.

- Include more soy foods – another good source of plant-based protein. Snack on dry roasted edamame, which you can buy in ready-to-eat packages in many supermarkets. Find a quality brand of soy burger to replace ground beef on your bun – looking for those proteins that have fewer artificial ingredients and more whole ingredients, such as vegetables, grains, and beans.

 Combine simmered whole grains, sautéed or raw vegetables, and cooked legumes on your plate. This age-old combination provides the perfect blend of proteins and nutrients to fuel your body.

STEP 4: LIMIT OTHER FOODS

Knowing which foods are less nutritious is just as important as understanding which foods are nutritious. If you follow these simple steps to healthy eating and reduce the foods containing less nutrition, you can ensure that you are on the right track.

SALT

Besides contributing to high blood pressure, consuming high amounts of sodium can also lead to stroke, heart disease, and heart failure.[1]

High blood pressure is a leading cause of cardiovascular disease. It accounts for two-thirds of all strokes and half of heart disease.[4]

80% of salt in the average diet is not from what you add in your kitchen or at the table, but what is contained in packaged, prepared, (restaurants) and processed foods. Avoiding processed foods is a key way to limit excess salt.

Harvard Health recommends reducing daily sodium intake to less than 2,300 milligrams to help control your blood pressure. Further reduction of sodium to no more than 1,500 milligrams per day may be beneficial for even better effects on blood pressure and is recommended for those who have high blood pressure (hypertension) or prehypertension.

SATURATED FAT

Saturated fats are a subject of recent debate; see the Fat section for more details. Though many research efforts are inconclusive, it is true that saturated fat increases harmful cholesterol (LDL). High cholesterol is one of the major risk factors for heart disease.[5]

Harvard Health recommends consuming less than 10% of calories from saturated fats. These fats are found in animal products such as butter, cream, cheese, fatty meats, and tropical oils such as palm, palm kernel, and coconut oil. Try replacing saturated fats with monounsaturated fats and polyunsaturated fats, such as vegetable oils, olives, nuts, seeds, and avocados. (Meat such as beef, pork, and lamb tends to be high in saturated fat, so it's best to limit your consumption of these. According to the American Institute for Cancer Research, you should also avoid cured and processed meats such as ham, sausage, and bacon).

ADDED SUGAR

Added sugars make up at least 10% of the calories that the average American eats in a day. But about one in 10 people get a whopping one-quarter or more of their calories from added sugar.[1] This excess sugar has a myriad of negative effects on our bodies including abdominal obesity, blood sugar levels, adrenal fatigue, (see our guide on Adrenal Fatigue: The 21st Century Stress Syndrome), hormone imbalance, and high blood pressure.

According to Harvard Health, over the course of the 15-year study, participants who took in 25% or more of their daily calories as sugar were more than twice as likely to die from heart disease as those whose diets included less than 10% added sugar. Overall, the odds of dying from heart disease rose in tandem with the percentage of sugar in the diet—and that was true regardless of a person's age, sex, physical activity level, and body-mass index (a measure of weight).

Harvard Health recommends that you limit added sugars to no more than 10% of total calories (about 50 grams to 12.5 teaspoons of sugar for the average person). Also, limit other refined foods (simple carbs that turn to sugar in the body) like white flour and white rice.

ALCOHOL

Drinking a lot of alcohol over a long period of time or too much on a single occasion can damage the heart, cause problems including stroke and high blood pressure, and negatively affect the liver, pancreas, and immune system. Drinking too much can weaken your immune system, making your body a much easier target for disease. High alcohol consumption can also increase your chances of certain cancers such as mouth, esophagus, throat, liver, and breast cancer.

Harvard Health recommends that, if you drink, do so in moderation, meaning no more than one drink per day for women and two drinks per day for men. Saving all your drinking for the weekend means that you take in unhealthy amounts of alcohol at a single sitting.

Those who are pregnant or under the legal drinking age should not drink at all.

ELIMINATE

Foods that you should eliminate are manufactured foods or non-foods, which are a product of man, and not nature.

ARTIFICIAL TRANS FAT

Trans fats raise your bad (LDL) cholesterol levels and lower your good (HDL) cholesterol levels. Eating trans fats increases your risk of developing heart disease and stroke. It's also associated with a higher risk of developing type 2 diabetes.

There are two broad types of trans fats found in foods: naturally occurring and artificial trans fats. Naturally occurring trans fats are produced in the gut of some animals, and foods made from these animals (e.g., milk and meat products) may contain small quantities of these fats. Artificial trans fats (or trans fatty acids) are created in an industrial process that adds hydrogen to liquid vegetable oils to make them more solid.

The primary dietary source of trans fats in processed food is "partially hydrogenated oils."

Eliminate artificial trans fats, such as those found in partially hydrogenated oils. In 2015, the FDA issued a ban on trans fats in processed foods, but manufacturers have until 2018 to comply; until then, it's worthwhile to check food labels for them. (see figure 2)

Because amounts less than 0.5 grams can be listed as 0, you should also check ingredient lists for partially hydrogenated vegetable oils.

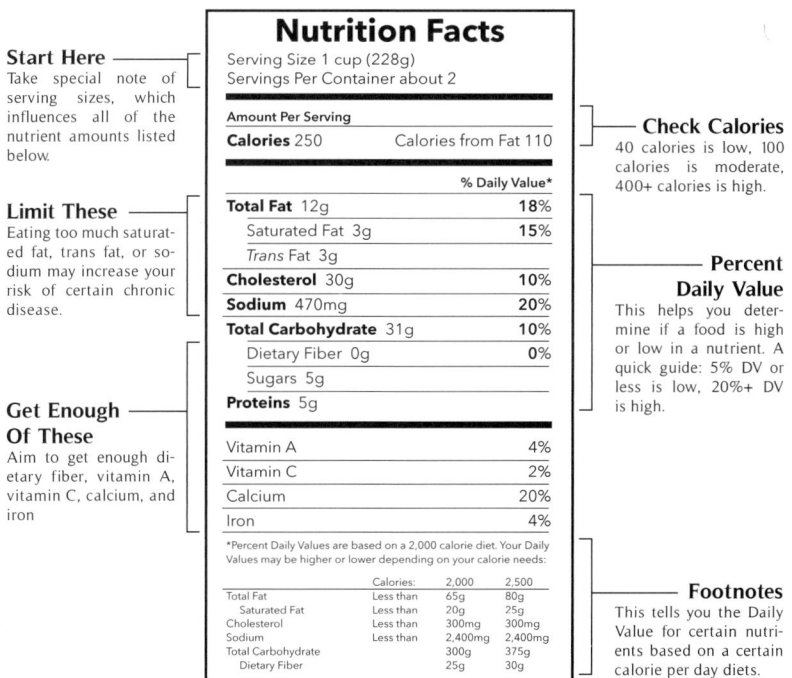

For the Love of Living

Chapter Three
THE SCIENCE OF FOOD

N ow that you know the principles of nutritious eating, you can begin to educate yourself on the qualities of food in order to make educated choices for yourself.

NUTRITION BASICS[6]

Nutrients can be divided into 2 categories: macronutrients and micronutrients. Macronutrients are those nutrients that the body needs in large amounts. These provide the body with energy (calories). Micronutrients are those nutrients that the body needs in smaller amounts.

MACRONUTRIENTS:
1. Carbohydrates
2. Proteins
3. Fats

MICRONUTRIENTS:
  WATER SOLUBLE VITAMINS
  - Vitamin B1
  - Vitamin B2
  - Vitamin B6
  - Vitamin B12
  - Vitamin C
  - Folic Acid

  FAT SOLUBLE VITAMINS
  - Vitamin A
  - Vitamin D
  - Vitamin E
  - Vitamin K

  MINERALS
  - Calcium
  - Potassium
  - Sodium
  - Iron
  - Zinc

  WATER

  PHYTOCHEMICALS

CARBOHYDRATES

Function:
1. Fuel during high-intensity exercise
2. Spares protein (to preserve muscle mass during exercise)
3. Fuel for the central nervous system (your brain)

Recommended Allowance:
1. Sedentary Individuals: 40-50% of your total daily calories should be carbohydrates

2. Exercises Regularly: 60% of your total daily calories should be carbohydrates
3. Athletes or persons involved in heavy training: 70% of your total daily calories should be carbohydrates (3.5-4.5 grams of carbohydrate per pound of body weight)

NOTE: 1 gram of carbohydrate = 4 Calories

Food Sources:
1. Grains (choose primarily whole grains for added benefits)
2. Dairy (choose low-fat or non-fat most often)
3. Fruit (choose whole fruits more often than fruit juices)

PROTEINS

Function:
1. Tissue structure (part of organ tissues, muscle, hair, skin, nails, bones, tendons, ligaments, and blood plasma)
2. Part of cell plasma membranes
3. Involved in metabolic, transport, and hormone systems
4. Make up enzymes that regulate metabolism
5. Involved in acid/base balance to maintain a neutral environment in our bodies

Recommended Allowance:
1. Sedentary Individuals: 0.36 grams of protein per pound of body weight
2. Recreationally Active: 045-0.68 grams of protein per pound of body weight
3. Competitive Athlete: 0.54-0.82 grams of protein per pound of body weight
4. Teenage Athlete: 0.82-0.91 grams of protein per pound of body weight
5. Body Builder: 0.64-0.91 grams of protein per pound of body weight

6. When restricting Calories: 0364-0.91 grams of protein per pound of body weight
7. Maximum amount of protein the body can utilize: 0.91 grams of protein per pound of body weight

NOTE: 1 gram of protein = 4 Calories

Food Sources:
1. Meat
2. Fish
3. Dairy
4. Legumes
5. Eggs

FATS

Function:
1. Energy reserve
2. Protects vital organs
3. Insulation
4. Transport fat soluble vitamins

Recommended Allowance:
1. 20-35% of your total daily calories should come from fat
2. Less than 10% of total daily calories should come from saturated fat (coconut and palm kernel oil, shortening, butter, cream, cheese, full-fat dairy products)

NOTE: 1 gram of fat = 9 Calories

Food Sources:
1. Oils
2. Nuts
3. Seeds
4. Meat, fish, dairy

VITAMIN B1: THIAMIN

Function:
1. Needed to release energy in food
2. Prevents beriberi – a disease resulting from lack of thiamin, which can affect the heart and the nervous system.

Food Sources:
1. Meat
2. Whole grains
3. Dried beans
4. Peas
5. Peanuts

VITAMIN B2: RIBOFLAVIN

Function:
1. Needed to build and maintain body tissue

Food Sources:
1. Organ meats
2. Meat
3. Eggs
4. Green and yellow vegetables
5. Enriched flour

VITAMIN B6: PYRIDOXINE

Function:
1. Helps the development of the nervous system
2. Involved in the production of blood
3. Helps break down protein and glucose to produce energy for the body

Food Sources:
1. Meats
2. Vegetables
3. Yeast
4. Nuts
5. Beans
6. Fish
7. Rice

VITAMIN B12: COBALAMINE

Function:
1. Promotes proper growth and developement of the nervous system

Food Sources:
1. Meats
2. Dairy
3. Eggs

VITAMIN C: ASCORBIC ACID

Function:
1. Helps form growth hormones
2. Needed to build strong gums, teeth, and bones
3. Antioxidant

Food Sources:
1. Citrus fruits
2. Cabbage
3. Berries
4. Peppers

FOLIC ACID

Function:
1. Helps build DNA and protein
2. Helps maintain intestinal tract
3. Aids in bone growth
4. Prevents nervous system birth defects

Food Sources:
1. Dark green leafy vegetables
2. Yeast
3. Wheat germ

VITAMIN A: RETINAL

Function:
1. Vision
2. Healthy skin
3. Healthy hair

Food Sources:
1. Milk
2. Butter
3. Margarine
4. Eggs
5. Cheese
6. Liver
7. Body can make vitamin A from vegetables that have carotene

VITAMIN D

Function:
1. Promotes strong teeth and bones
2. Prevents rickets - a disorder resulting from a lack of vitamin D, calcium, or phosphate, which lead to a softening and weakening of the bones.

Food Sources:
1. Milk
2. Cod liver oil
3. Tuna
4. Salmon
5. Egg yolks
6. Produced by the body when exposed to sunlight

VITAMIN E

Function:
1. Prevents damage to cell membranes
2. Protects vitamin A
3. Aids in blood production

Food Sources:
1. Seeds and nuts
2. Vegetable oil

VITAMIN K

Function:
1. Aids in blood clotting

Food Sources:
1. Green leafy vegetables
2. Produced by bacteria in the large intestine

CALCIUM

Function:
1. Maintains teeth and bones
2. Helps blood to clot
3. Helps nerves and muscles function

Food Sources:
1. Cheese
2. Milk
3. Dark green vegetables
4. Sardines
5. Clams
6. Oysters
7. Legumes

POTASSIUM

Function:
1. Regulates water balance in cells
2. Helps nerves function
3. Important for heart rhythm

Food Sources:
1. Oranges
2. Bananas
3. Meats
4. Poultry
5. Fish
6. Cereal
7. Potatoes
8. Dried beans

SODIUM

Function:
1. Regulates water balance
2. Stimulates nerves

Food Sources:
1. Table salt
2. Meat
3. Poultry
4. Fish
5. Eggs
6. Milk

IRON

Function:
1. Forms blood cells
2. Transports oxygen throughout the body

Food Sources:
1. Liver
2. Red meats
3. Dark green vegetables
4. Whole-grain cereals
5. Shellfish

ZINC

Function:
1. Aids in transport of carbon dioxide
2. Aids in healing wounds
3. Forms enzymes

Food Sources:
1. Meats
2. Shellfish
3. Whole grains
4. Milk
5. Legumes

The Science of Food

PHYTOCHEMICALS

"Plant Chemicals" - Compounds with antioxidant and anti-inflammatory effects. See Vitamins, Minerals, & Phytochemicals in Understanding Nutrition to find out more.

WATER

Function:
1. Moistens tissues such as those in the mouth, eyes, and nose
2. Protects body organs and tissues
3. Helps prevent constipation
4. Helps dissolve minerals and other nutrients to make them accessible to the body
5. Regulates body temperature
6. Lubricates joints
7. Lessens the burden on the kidneys and liver by flushing out waste products
8. Carries nutrients and oxygen to cells

CARBOHYDRATES

Carbs have acquired a bad reputation from current trends including the Paleo and Atkins diet as well as the gluten-free trend, which is only intended for those with celiac disease and gluten-sensitivity.

Carbohydrate-rich foods are vital to your health. **Carbohydrates are an important macronutrient that provide your body with a source of energy to fuel your daily activities.** Many carb-containing foods like whole grains, vegetables, fruits, and legumes are rich in other nutrients that your body needs including fiber, vitamins, and minerals. If you significantly reduce your intake of these carbs, it will be hard for you to get these nutrients that your body needs.

The AMDR (acceptable macronutrient distribution ranges) recommends that your **daily intake of carbohydrates make up 40-65% of your diet.** By including fruits, vegetables, and whole grains at each meal and snack, you will easily achieve this level of healthy carbs.

DID YOU KNOW?: Fruits and vegetables contain carbs. Carbs are a macronutrient your body needs for energy.

Rather than avoiding carbs altogether, it is a better solution to choose healthier carbs.

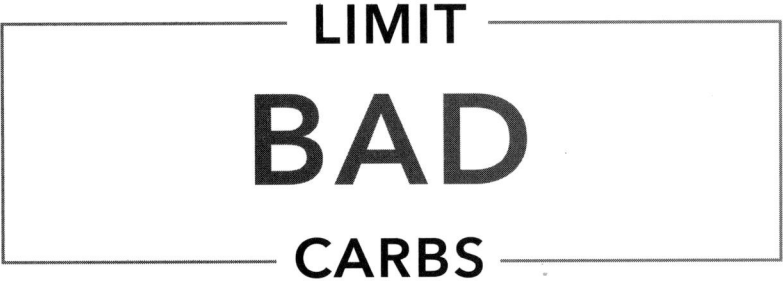

The carbs to avoid are those in processed foods. That includes foods made out of refined grains (such as white pasta and snacks) and refined sugars (such as sweetened beverages, desserts, and baked goods). These types of carbs are:

Simple Carbohydrates – Your body turns these carbs to sugar much faster, and they impair the body's ability to manage blood glucose levels, causing blood sugar spikes. This will leave you feeling hungry and void of energy and will encourage the storage of fat.

These carbohydrates are void of nutrition. A diet high in simple carbs can lead to diabetes, heart disease, kidney problems, obesity, and cancer.

CHOOSE GOOD CARBS

Make most of your carb choices from whole or minimally processed carb-rich foods, such as whole grains, legumes, vegetables, and fruits. These carbs are:

Complex Carbohydrates – Absorb more slowly in the body giving you longer lasting energy and keep you feeling more full, longer.

These carbohydrates are packed with healthy fiber, vitamins, minerals, and phytochemicals. A diet with the recommend dosage of complex carbs can reduce the risk of heart disease.

WHOLE GRAINS

Whole grains have an incredible number of benefits for our health, including reduced risk of cardiovascular disease, type 2 diabetes, and colorectal cancer. Why are these simple plant foods - especially the seed of grasses - so protective? Harvard Health says that one reason is that the fiber-rich outer covering called bran slows the breakdown of starch into glucose and helps the body maintain a steady blood sugar level. Fiber also helps lower cholesterol and move food through the digestive tract. The embryo, or germ, is equally important, containing a wealth of vitamins and minerals, as you'll realize if you read the Nutrition Facts on a package of wheat germ. Among these nutrients are essential B-vitamins and minerals like magnesium, selenium, and copper. If you were to completely eliminate whole grains from your diet - as some fads suggest - you'd fall short on many key nutrients needed for optimal health.

FIBER

Fiber is another reason why a diet rich in good carbs is so healthy. Fiber does many useful things while it's in your digestive tract, such as:

- Slows down digestion and lowers a food's glycemic index value, a measure of how quickly the sugar in the food enters your bloodstream.

- Causes you to feel full for a longer period of time, helping control appetite and weight gain.

- Slightly reduces "bad" LDL cholesterol

- Reduces insulin resistance

- Promotes bowel health

As with other nutrients, fiber is best when taken in from whole foods rather than processed ones. Beware of "added isolated fiber" such as inulin added to many foods in order to increase the total volume of fiber. Though insulin has been shown to have some benefits related to nourishing friendly gut bacteria, it is not linked to the multitude of health benefits found in foods that are naturally rich in fiber such as oranges, berries, almonds, lentils, flaxseed, and other whole grains.

GREAT CHOICES OF WHOLE GRAIN

Remember to eat a variety of whole grains to enjoy all the nutritional benefits they offer.

- **Amaranth** - Mild flavor. Rich in calcium and iron. Naturally gluten-free and good in hot cereal, added to rice, or ground into whole-grain flour for baking.

- **Barley** - A crunchy grain rich in a type of fiber called beta-glucans, barley has special heart health benefits related to its ability to lower blood cholesterol levels. Great in soups, casseroles, salads, and as a side dish.

- **Buckwheat** - Naturally gluten-free (not a true wheat, but a cousin to rhubarb). The nutty flavor is great in pancakes, in salads, side dishes, or soups.

- **Millet** - A small grain that is great cooked in cereals and desserts, and is ground into flour for breads such as Indian roti.

- **Sorghum** - Can be served as a hot cereal, ground into flour for bread, or even popped like popcorn.

- **Oats** - When eaten daily, oats have been linked to significantly lower blood cholesterol levels. Beyond the breakfast table, oats can be added to breads, fruit-based desserts, and meals like risotto.

- **Quinoa** - High in nutritional value. Mild flavored and quick-cooking, it is great in side dishes, salads, and as a filling for vegetables.

- **Rice** - Brown colored (including black, purple, or red) and wild rice are all whole grains (although wild rice is not a true rice). As a mild-tasting grain, it is great with savory foods.

- **Rye** - A standard feature in breads, rye is also good steamed and served as a hot cereal, in side dishes, and as a filling for vegetables.

- **Teff** - For it's tiny, poppy-seed like size, teff is packed with nutrients. Great in cereals, grain side dishes, and baked goods.

- **Wheat** - Best known as a flour but also comes in the forms of bulgur, faro, spelt, and wheat berries.

For the Love of Living

IDENTIFYING WHOLE GRAINS IN FOOD YOU BUY:
Food items advertised as whole grain do not always meet the requirements to qualify them as actually whole grain. A true whole grain should contain **at least 3 grams of fiber** per serving. You can check the nutritional facts for information and also look for the Old-Ways Whole Grains Council stamp.

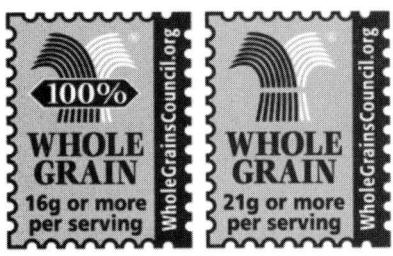

If a product bears the 100% Stamp (shown on the left), then all its grain ingredients are whole grains. There is a minimum requirement of 16g (16 grams) – a full serving – of whole grain per labeled serving, for products using the 100% Stamp.

If a product bears the Basic Stamp (shown on the right), it contains at least 8g (8 grams) – a half serving – of whole grain, but may also contain some refined grain. Even if a product contains significant amounts of whole grain (23g, 37g, 41g, etc.), it will use the Basic Stamp if it also contains extra bran, germ, or refined flour.

Photo Credit: The Whole Grains Council

ADDED SUGAR
Added sugar refers to the sugar that is not naturally occurring in food like fruit or carrots, but the kind extracted from sugar cane and beets then added to foods. As it has addictive qualities, sugar has been described as a drug, which explains why it is that the more you eat, the more you want.

Added sugar lacks nutritional value but has increased calories, and with its addictive qualities, is a leading cause of the problem with obesity in the US. Unfortunately, corporations use this sugar addiction as a way to increase their profits, to the detriment of our

The Science of Food

CARBS

Daily diet:
45% - 60%
48g

MACRONUTRIENTS TO FUEL ENERGY

BAD CARBS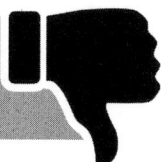

 ### GOOD CARBS

REFINED SUGAR
Table sugar
High fructose corn syrup
Honey

REFINED FLOUR
Breads
Bagels
Baked Goods

DESSERTS, ICE CREAM
Pastries
Beverages
Sweetened yogurt
Sugary cereals

HIGH GLYCEMIC
Potatoes
White rice
Fruit Juice

PROCESSED "QUICK"
Quick oats
Quick grits

PROCESSED REFINED GRAINS WHITE SUGARS

- Stripped of nutrients
- Blood sugar spikes
- Store fat
- Diabetes, heart desease, kidney problems, obesity, cancer

WHOLE GRAIN
A N A T O M Y

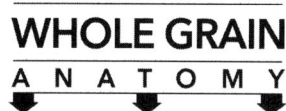

Endosperm —
Bran
Germ

FIBER HELPS WITH
- Slowing breakdown of sugar/digestion
- Feeling Fuller
- Bowel health
- Reducing bad cholesterol

WHOLE GRAINS

LEGUMES, VEGGIES, FRUIT

+ Fiber, vitamins, minerals, phytochemicals

+ Reduced risk of health issues

- Amaranth
- Barley
- Buckwheat
- Millet
- Oats
- Quinoa   • Sorghum
- Rice   • Teff
- Rye   • Wheat

HOW TO TELL

Whole grain listed 1st in ingredients

At least 3g of fiber

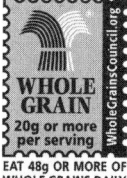

EAT 48g OR MORE OF WHOLE GRAINS DAILY

FIBER

MEN: 38g - WOMEN: 25g

*Beware of added isolated fiber

health. You'll find sugar, including processed high-fructose sugars, in products that you wouldn't expect to have sugar at all, such as canned tomato soup.

So how can we still enjoy the sweet things we love without going overboard? The Dietary Guidelines recommend limiting added sugar to 10% of your calories — about 200 calories or 50 grams (12.5 teaspoons) of added sugar each day for the average person. It is easy to exceed this recommendation when eating processed foods, so you will be much more successful when enjoying your food in it's whole or minimally processed form. Limit packaged foods, prepared foods (restaurants), baked goods, and fast foods.

Hidden Sugar
Inspect the ingredient list for added sugar in foods like breakfast cereals, granola bars, canned soups, and yogurt. Added sugars are frequently found in such items, and they turn out to be much more like a dessert than a nutritious meal.

Natural Sugars
Note that while "natural" sugars, such as agave, coconut palm sugar, and honey are less processed than cane or beet sugar and are growing in popularity, they still are added sugars and should be limited.

FATS

In the past, people were reluctant to include fat in their diet because they thought that consuming it is what caused them to gain weight. In reality, the body only stores fat when increased insulin from sugar consumption is in your bloodstream. Fat is an essential macronutrient that has many beneficial qualities for our health. It is a primary source of energy that helps fuel your daily activity, insulates your body, and keeps you warm. Your body requires fat to make cell membranes, sheath the nerves, maintain healthy skin and hair, and perform other vital functions. It aids in the absorption of certain key nutrients from your diet, such as the fat-soluble vitamins A, D, E, and K, and it also plays the much-appreciated role of making our food taste better.

You should aim to get 20-35% of your daily calories from fat – about 44-78 grams for the average person.

Rather than avoiding fat altogether, we can choose the types of fat that are healthier for us.

GOOD FATS
In general, the good fats come from plant sources and fish and are liquid at room temperature, while bad fats come from animal or man-made sources and are solid at room temperature.

Polyunsaturated Fats - Polyunsaturated fats are fats that our bodies do not produce on their own, therefore they are essential to the diet. They are required for normal body functions including brain development, inflammation control, and blood clotting. The two principal sources of polyunsaturated fats are omega3 fatty acids and omega-6 fatty acids, which are found in fish oil, flaxseeds, and sunflower seeds.

> **Omega 3 Fatty Acid** – This nutrient helps prevent and treat heart disease and stroke, reduces blood pressure, lowers triglycerides, and helps prevent heart rhythm disorders. It also raises HDL (good) cholesterol. **Sources:** Fatty fish such as salmon, mackerel, and sardines are the best. Also found in flaxseeds, walnuts, canola oil, and soy.
>
> *Although you can take omega-3 as a supplement, research shows that it is more effective to receive this nutrient through your food.*
>
> **Omega 6 Fatty Acid** – Research shows evidence of protec-

tion from heart disease, and helping to lower levels of LDL (bad) cholesterol. **Sources:** Vegetable oils such as safflower, soybean, sunflower, walnut, and corn oil.

Uses: Sautéing, salad dressing, baking

Monounsaturated Fats - Decrease the risk of cardiovascular disease and type 2 diabetes because they help improve blood cholesterol levels and your body's responsiveness to insulin. **Sources:** Olive oil, olives, canola oil, avocados, most nuts (along with their oils) safflower and sunflower oils.

BAD FATS

As stated above, the fat that is not as good for you comes from animal or man-made sources and is solid at room temperature. This includes,

Trans Fat - Although some trans fats occur naturally at very low levels in foods such as meat and dairy, health experts are mainly concerned with those that are man-made in the form of **partially-hydrogenated oil.** Because of the recent attention to this bad fat, it is being removed from foods; however, it can still be found in foods such as crackers, cookies, cakes, snack foods, stick margarine, coffee creamers, refrigerated dough products and ready-to-use frostings.

Trans fat holds no nutritional value and boosts the chances of developing heart disease by increasing blood levels of LDL (bad) cholesterol and triglycerides. Trans fat also has lower levels of protective HDL cholesterol, which make them even more harmful to your health.

The Science of Food

FATS

Daily diet:
20% - 35%
49g - 78g

SOURCE OF ENERGY & INSULATION - MACRONUTRIENT

BAD FATS

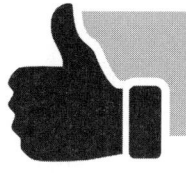

GOOD FATS

So what about **BUTTER & DAIRY?**
IT'S IN BETWEEN

+ Prevent heart disease
+ Inflamation control
+ Brain development

SOLID | At room temperature

LIQUID | At room temperature

SATURATED
animal foods

POLYUNSATURATED
(e s s e n t i a l)

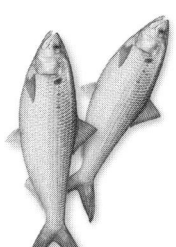

» Increases "bad" LDL cholestrol which effects heart health
» Evidence is inconclusive, but still a good idea to *keep low* & replace with polyunsaturated fats
» Heart Disease
• High-fat meats
• High-fat dairy (cheese, butter, whole milk, cream
• Tropical fats (palm oil, coconut oil)

Fish Oil •
Flaxseeds •
Sunflower Seeds •
Omega-3 Fatty Acid •
Omega-6 Fatty Acid •

MONOSATURATED

Olive Oil •
Canola Oil •
Avacodo •
Nuts •

TRANS FAT
mostly artificial | manufactured
• Partially hydrogenated oils
• Crackers, cookies, cakes, frozen pies
• Margarine, coffee creamer, processed and fried foods

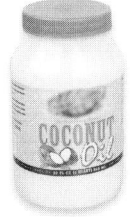

The hype about COCONUT OIL?
Saturated Fat. Keep Low.

LESS HEALTHFUL FATS
Saturated Fat - Saturated fats have been the subject of much debate. They can be found in animal products such as butter, whole milk, cream, high-fat meats and cheese, as well as in palm and coconut oil. There is inconclusive evidence that saturated fat has a negative effect on heart health. Experts at Harvard suggest that, in light of this data, you still limit saturated fats in your diet. The Dietary Guidelines, which are based on the entire body of evidence, recommend that saturated fat intake remains below 10% of dietary calories – about 22 grams per day for the average person. Research has shown that saturated fat elevates harmful LDL (bad) cholesterol.

COCONUT OIL
Did you know that although coconut oil has become very popular recently – being said to have all sorts of benefits such as "burning" fat, killing viruses, lowering cholesterol, and reducing seizures - there is little evidence to back up these claims. Coconut oil becomes solid at room temperature because it is 90% saturated fat, which raises LDL (bad) cholesterol. It has been pointed out that almost half of the saturated fat in coconut oil comes in the form of lauric acid, which boosts HDL (good) cholesterol. Because of the lack of supporting data, however, Harvard Health states that it is best to use it sparingly and go with healthier vegetable oils, such as olive and soybean oil.

PROTEIN
Protein is an essential part of our diet with multiple functions such as building the enzymes that trigger many of the body's vital chemical reactions. A lack of protein in the diet can slow growth, reduce muscle mass, lower immunity, weaken the heart and respiratory system, and even cause death. However, few Americans fall short of the necessary protein requirement.

Just like the other two macronutrients, there are good and not-so-good choices of protein. When choosing, you'll want to consider what else you'll find in the source of protein; does the food contain an unhealthy amount of saturated fat, like that found in ground beef, or does it come, as lentils do, with a healthy bonus of vitamins, minerals, and phytochemicals?

Amino Acids - Amino acids are the building blocks of protein. Although there are 20 amino acids, only 9 are considered essential to the body. Like the essential fats, these are the components the body cannot synthesize and must take in from food. Proponents of meat-heavy diets claim that meat is the superior source of protein because it is a "high-quality" protein containing significant amounts of all 9 essential amino acids. Harvard experts, however, state that you can get all of the essential amino acids by eating a variety of plant foods, such as legumes, soy, and nuts.

Healthful Protein - A majority of the most nutritious sources of protein are found in plant sources, fish, and poultry.

- **Legumes** – Dried beans, lentils, and peas. Rich in protein (about 8 grams per half cup, cooked) as well as fiber, folate, manganese, potassium, iron, magnesium, copper, selenium, zinc, and phytochemicals. Studies have shown that a diet rich in legumes is linked to lower risk of heart disease, hypertension, obesity, and some types of cancer and diabetes.

- **Soy** – (A part of the legume family), is a super food. Found in: Tofu, tempeh, soybeans, soy milk and soy nuts. It is uniquely rich in high-quality protein (about 15 grams per half cup, cooked) as well as iron, calcium and – in minimally processed forms – fiber. According to Harvard Health, soy also possesses phytoestrogens, which have antioxidant properties that may account for some of soy's health benefits, such as lower risk of heart disease. They also state that there is no reason to worry about the hype on the dangers of soy. There is no scientific basis for avoiding this wholesome food in its whole form in moderate amounts, which is 23 servings per day.

- **Nuts & Seeds** – From almonds to walnuts and from chia to sunflower, nuts and seeds are packed with plant-based protein (3-9 grams of protein per ounce, depending on the variety) as well as healthy fats, fiber, vitamins, minerals, and phytochemicals. Research shows that up to a handful of nuts and seeds a day can help lower heart disease.

- **Fish** – One of the best animal proteins you can choose. The American Heart Association suggests that you include at least two 3-ounce servings of fish or seafood in your diet weekly. Fish is high in protein and long chain omega3 fatty acids with benefits such as reduced risks of heart attacks, strokes, prostate cancer, depression, and Alzheimer's disease. It's important to be aware of mercury in fish and try to avoid those fish with the highest levels. Fish that is low in mercury include shrimp, canned light tuna, salmon, pollock, and catfish.

- **Poultry** – The second best choice of animal protein is skinless chicken and turkey, which provide a good source of protein with minimal saturated fat.

RED MEAT

Red meat is a favorite comfort food among many cultures. There is nothing wrong with enjoying an occasional steak; in fact, red meat carries a hefty dose of protein and also minerals, such as iron and zinc. However, several major studies indicate that diets heavy in red meat may contribute to a higher risk of disease. Harvard researchers have found that people who eat the most red meat tend to die at a younger age, with the cause of death commonly being heart disease and cancer. A contributing factor to these deaths may be the

The Science of Food

PROTEIN

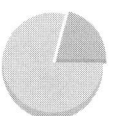

Daily diet:
10% - 35%
50g - 115g

MACRONUTRIENTS TO BUILD & MAINTAIN
AMERICANS TEND TO OVERESTIMATE HOW MUCH PROTEIN THEY NEED.

BAD PROTEIN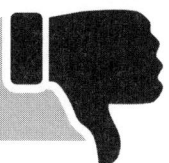

GOOD PROTEIN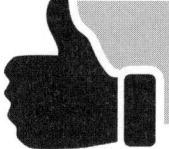

REMOVE MEAT AS YOUR MAIN SOURCE OF PROTEIN
ALL WHOLE FOODS CONTAIN PROTEIN
Protein deficiency is rare in the U.S.

- Maintain muscles, bone, skin & every other organ & tissue
- Build enzymes that trigger important chemical reactions
- Diet high in protein is usually lower in refined carbs

LIMIT: RED MEAT
- High in saturated fat, sodium » **Heart Disease**
- Cooked at high temperatures » **Cancer**

CHOOSE: Lean Cuts & Grass-fed Beef

PROCESSED MEAT
- Bacon, hot dogs, bologna, pepperoni » Group 1 carcinogen » **Colon cancer, heart disease, stroke, diabetes**

PLANT SOURCES
LEGUMES: beans, lentils, peas
» fiber, vitamins & minerals

SOY: tofu, tempeh, soybeans
» iron, calcium, fiber
(non-processed)

NUTS & SEEDS: almonds to pumpkin
» good fats, fiber, vitamins & minerals

ANIMAL SOURCES
FISH: fatty fish & seafood
» omega 3 fatty acid

POULTRY: chicken, turkey
» low saturated fat

DAIRY
- Protein & calcium
  BONE HEALTH
- Inconclusively linked to CERTAIN CANCERS (prostate, ovarian). Insulin-like growth factor in cows' milk.
  - Whole milk
  - Cottage Cheese
  - Ice Cream
» Limit to 2 low fat servings / Day
  + Milk
  + Cottage Cheese
  + Yogurt

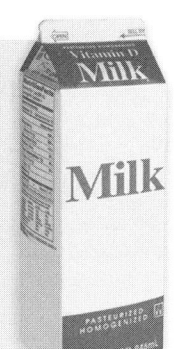

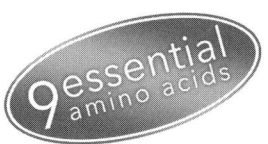

9 essential amino acids

Don't stress too much about getting these. You can usually get them through a variety of plant foods.

GRAINS + LEGUMES
rice + dahl (lentils)
rice + beans

| Soy has ALL 9

high levels of saturated fat found in many red meats. Your best bet is to limit red meat in your diet, replacing it with healthier forms of protein such as legumes and fish. When you do enjoy red meat, choose leaner options containing less than 2 grams of saturated fat per 3.5 ounces and limit your intake of cooked lean meat to no more than 6 ounces a day.

Cooking red meat at high temperatures, such as on the grill, promotes the formation of substances called heterocyclic amines, which can contribute to the development of cancer.

Processed Meat - The most unhealthy variety of meats are processed meats such as bacon, ham, hot dogs, bologna, salami, sausage, and pepperoni. Meat is qualified as "processed" is when it is "transformed through salting, curing, fermentation, smoking or other processes to enhance flavor or improve preservation." In 2015, the World Health Organization deemed processed meat as a Group 1 Carcinogen (raising the risk of cancer – specifically colon cancer in this case).

DAIRY

Dairy products such as milk, cheese, and yogurt are very nourishing and are excellent sources of the protein and calcium that are essential for bone health. While dairy has been linked to lowering the risk of colorectal cancer, there is also inconclusive research that dairy plays a part in prostate and ovarian cancers due to an insulin-like growth factor found in cow's milk and products made from whole milk, such as cottage cheese and ice cream. For these reasons, it's a good idea to limit dairy consumption and choose low-fat varieties when you do have it. A great alternate source of calcium are green, leafy vegetables, broccoli, and beans.

VITAMINS, MINERALS & PHYTOCHEMICALS

Just like the macronutrients (carbs, fat, and protein), your body needs vitamins and minerals to fuel the growth and life happening inside of you. Though your body only needs a small amount of micronutrients, falling short can be detrimental to your health. British sailors who were out at sea for months at a time without fresh fruits and vegetables realized that a lack of vitamin C led to scurvy – which often was fatal.

So, how do you know if you're getting enough? The best answer is the same as the one for most other nutrition questions – eat a well-rounded diet with a variety of colors and types of whole foods, especially plants, along with healthy fats such as nuts and olive oil.

SUPPLEMENTS

In most cases, it is better to get your vitamins and minerals from your diet rather than supplements. If you are falling short, however, a supplement may be necessary.

According to Harvard Health, one problem with taking supplements of the fat-soluble vitamins (A, D, E, and K) is that they are not readily passed through the body – unlike the water-soluble vitamins (C and B), which are excreted in the urine if they're not needed. If the body does not use the fat-soluble vitamins, they are stored in fat and can build up to toxic levels if taken too frequently. In contrast, you are unlikely to get too many vitamins and minerals from food in its natural form. For this reason, it is better to take fewer supplements and observe the dosage recommendation when you do.

SHORTFALL NUTRIENTS

It is more difficult to obtain your daily quota of the following nutrients, so more attention has to be given to procuring them:

Potassium – Daily Recommendations: 4,700 mg. You can boost intake by adding more fruits, vegetables, and beans to diet. Bananas, citrus, avocados, kiwi, and melon are great sources.

Calcium – Daily Recommendation: 1,000 mg. You can boost your intake by including dairy, yogurt, or calcium-fortified non-dairy milk twice a day. Dark green, leafy vegetables are also a good source of calcium, such as kale, bok choy, broccoli, and spinach.

Vitamin D – Daily Recommendation: 600 IU (International Units). 5-10 minutes a day of unprotected sun exposure on the hands, arms, and legs can provide vitamin D. Fish that are rich in fats such as salmon, sardines, mackerel, rainbow trout, and tuna are also an excellent source, as are fortified dairy products.

Dietary Fiber – Daily Recommendation: 21-38 grams. You can boost your intake by replacing most of the refined grains that you eat with whole grains.

ANTIOXIDANTS

Antioxidants are your body's natural defense against intruders or free radicals (damaging chemicals formed from metabolism, the environment, and even the sun). While everyone needs antioxidants, it has become the latest craze in the media, with laboratories advertising the content of fruits, vegetables, herbs, and spices and presenting number values of antioxidant rich foods. However, according to Harvard Health, these sources have over-simplified the idea. It is important to realize that antioxidants from different sources serve different purposes. For instance, the beta-carotene in carrots quenches a particularly damaging free radical called superoxide. In contrast, the vitamin E in nuts and avocados is rela-

VITAMINS • MINERALS
PHYTOCHEMICALS
MICRONUTRIENTS TO ORCHESTRATE & SUSTAIN LIFE

ANTIOXIDANTS
- Fight off free-radicals that come from metabolism, environment & the sun

WHY ANTIOXIDANT PROMOS ON STORE FOOD AREN'T ALWAYS EFFECTIVE
- Some need to work together
- Processing destroys some antioxidants
- Some perform differently in the lab than in the body

GET ANTIOXIDANTS THROUGH FRESH FRUITS & VEGETABLES
- Best option, even though some antioxidants found in fruits & veggies deteriorate over time.

PHYTOCHEMICALS
"PLANT CHEMICALS" NOT ONLY BENEFIT PLANTS, BUT US TOO!
- Lutein (dark leafy veg.) - **Helps prevent eye ailments**
- Lycopene (tomatoes) - **Prostate disease defense**
- Proanthocyanidins (cranberries) - **UTI**
- Sulphoraphane (cruciferous veg.) - **Fights cancer**

VEGETABLES
- Choose a variety of colors

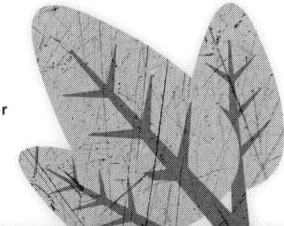

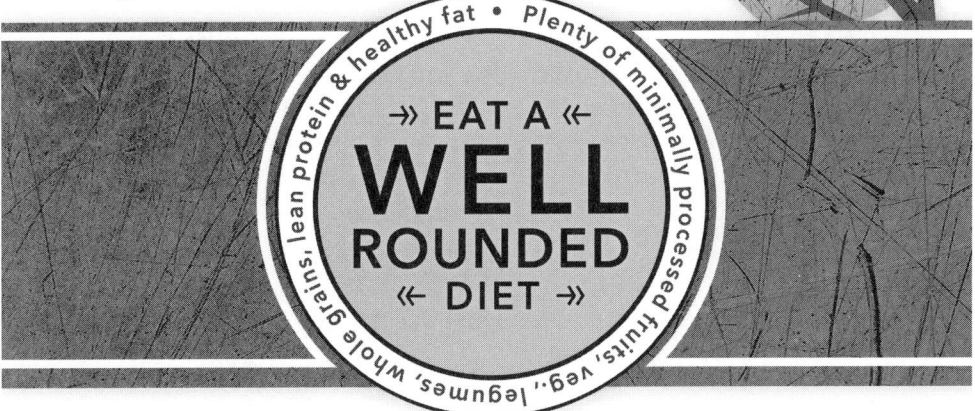

→ EAT A ←
WELL ROUNDED
← DIET →

healthy fat • Plenty of minimally processed fruits, veg., legumes, whole grains, lean protein &

THE BODY ALSO PRODUCES ANTIDIOXIDANTS...
... But focus primarily on your diet.

FOOD vs. SUPPLEMENTS
- Evidence in tests shows supplements to be less effective
- Too many supplements can be taken

SHORTFALL NUTRIENTS
- Potassium
- Calcium
- Vitamin D
- Dietary Fiber

ARE YOU GETTING ENOUGH?
You can track this, but don't stress over it. Just eat a well-rounded diet.

tively powerless against superoxide – though it serves the equally important function of bolstering LDL (bad) cholesterol against oxidation. This helps reduce the chance of heart attack. Antioxidants also operate in networks, meaning some of them need other ones to work effectively. It is best to get antioxidants through a variety of whole foods rather than those added to processed foods, because processing destroys certain antioxidants. Even for whole foods with antioxidant ratings, some perform differently in lab tests than in the body. According to Harvard Health, the bottom line is: Eating a variety of colorful plant foods is a good thing - just don't get too caught up in their antioxidant content.

PHYTOCHEMICALS

Phytochemicals or "plant chemicals" are compounds found in plants that aid in their development, such as the color, flavor, and scent of foods like tomatoes, garlic, and oranges.

These chemicals have wonderful benefits for us as well. There are thousands of phytochemicals in your fruits and vegetables and in many cases they work in networks, so taking them in supplement form is not as effective as having them in your diet. Here are a few.

> **Lutein** (Found in dark, leafy vegetables) - protect against specific eye ailments
>
> **Lycopene** (Found in tomatoes) - provides defense against prostate disease
>
> **Proanthocyanidins** (Found in cranberries) - wards off urinary track infections
>
> **Sulforaphane** (Found in cruciferous vegetables – plants with four-petaled flowers) - fight cancer by mopping up certain cancer-promoting substances that form in your body during normal metabolism.

LIQUIDS

Of all the ways that we can consume calories, doing so in liquid form is the easiest. We can also think we are hungry when we are, in fact, thirsty. Water is the most essential liquid that we can consume, and we should have a certain amount every day to aid certain critical functions. Follow this guideline for daily liquid intake.

WATER
DID YOU KNOW? The Brain is 73% water. Optimal brain function depends on water and lots of it; that's what keeps the brain signals going. According to H.H. Mitchell, Journal of Biological Chemistry 158, the brain and heart are composed of 73% water, and the lungs are about 83% water. The skin contains 64% water, muscles and kidneys are 79%, and even the bones contain water: 31%7

Daily Recommendation: 13 - 8oz. servings for men I 9 - 8oz. servings for women (The amount needed depends on a number of factors including your size, activity level, and the weather).

Water plays an incredibly important role in the body, which is why it's best for most of your liquid intake to be water. Some of the benefits are:

- Aids in digestion

- Prevents constipation

- Normalizes blood pressure

- Stabilizes heartbeat

- Carries nutrients and oxygen to cells

- Cushions joints

- Protects organs and tissues

- Helps regulate body temperature

- Maintains electrolyte balance

COFFEE & TEA
Coffee and tea are your second-best choices of liquids, after water. They are both derived from plants and are packed with antioxidant and anti-inflammatory elements. They also contain caffeine, which aids in alertness and performance. *Note: Adding sugar and milk can make these drinks a less healthy choice.

LIMIT OR AVOID
Drinks to limit or avoid include sugary beverages, which are an easy way to consume excess calories; it's easier to consume more calories in a liquid than in food.

Sugary Beverages - Sugary beverages are the leading source of added sugar in the American diet and linked to obesity, type 2 diabetes, and heart disease. It is the top provider of calories in the American diet.

- **Soft Drinks** – A can of pop contains about 35 grams of added sugar.

- **Sports Drinks** – Water has been proven to be the best fuel for activity; these sugary drinks are not necessarily helpful to your performance in the long run.

- **Energy Drinks** – The extremely high caffeine content can have a negative effect on your health.

- **Juice Drinks** – Many juice drinks have added sugar. Even those without added sugar contain a highly concentrated amount of natural sugar (it takes many more oranges to make a glass of juice than you'd usually eat whole). Limit juice to one serving a day.

LIQUIDS

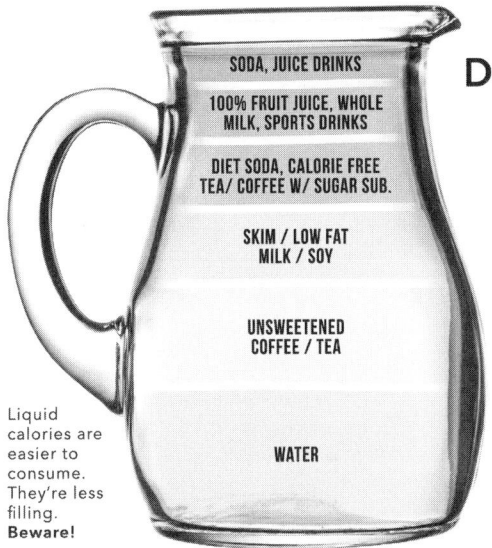

SODA, JUICE DRINKS

100% FRUIT JUICE, WHOLE MILK, SPORTS DRINKS

DIET SODA, CALORIE FREE TEA/ COFFEE W/ SUGAR SUB.

SKIM / LOW FAT MILK / SOY

UNSWEETENED COFFEE / TEA

WATER

Liquid calories are easier to consume. They're less filling. **Beware!**

WOMEN: 9 CUPS OF WATER / DAY
MEN: 13 CUPS OF WATER / DAY

DRINK *MORE* WATER

PHYSICAL BENEFITS
- Aids in digestion
- Prevents constipation
- Normalizes blood pressure
- Stabilizes heart beat
- Carries nutrients and O^2 to cells
- Cushions joints
- Protects organs & tissues
- Helps regulate body temp.
- Maintains electrolyte balance
- 70% of brain fuel
- 80% of muscle fuel

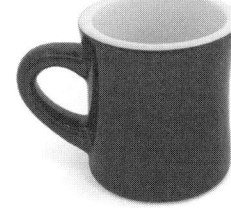

Can be helpful, but it's still best to rely on your diet for vitamins and antioxidants.

LIMIT:

SUGARY BEVERAGES
LEADING SOURCE OF ADDED SUGAR IN DIETS
- Linked to obesity, type 2 heart diabetes & heart disease
- Top providers of calories in diets

JUICE DRINKS
- More natural sugar
- Processing removes much, if not all fiber
- Avoid added sugar

ALCOHOL
- Poses risk to liver, heart health and increases risk of breast cancer.
» If you enjoy it: **Moderate** | If not: **Avoid**

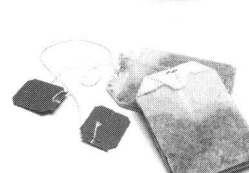

COFFEE & TEA
- 2nd best to water
- Antidioxidants & anti-inflammatory, plant-derived caffeine
- Tea: heart health, cancer defense, immune function, bone health, weight loss.
Beware:
- Extra calories
- Caffeine has a negative effect on some people
- Bottled Tea

Alcohol - Some sources may proclaim red wine a health tonic, but Harvard Health says the science is a bit more confusing. Moderate consumption of alcohol, not just red wine, has been linked to heart health benefits (no more than one serving a day for women and 2 for men). However, there are several risks involved. These include a range of health problems such as liver and heart disease as well as certain cancers like breast, colon, mouth, throat, and esophageal cancer. If you enjoy drinking alcohol, do so in moderation; if you do not currently drink, the benefits are not significant enough to take up the habit.

The Science of Food

OVERVIEW

FOCUS

PLANTS
- Fruit
- Vegetables
- Legumes
- Soy
- Nuts, seeds
- Whole grains

FISH
FERMENTED FOODS
BLACK / GREEN TEA
BLUEBERRIES
BROCCOLI
EGGS
NUTS
ORANGES
OATMEAL
BLACK BEANS
SPINACH/ KALE
AVACADO
SALMON
E.V. OLIVE OIL
QUINOA
DARK CHOCOLATE
TOMATOES
TURKEY

AVOID

REFINED/WHITE
- Sugar
- Flour
- High-fructose corn syrup

TRANS FAT
- Partially hydrogenated oils

BOXED
PACKAGED
DRIVE-THRU

LIMIT

SATURATED FATS
HIGH-FAT DAIRY
- Whole milk
- Cheese
- Butter
- Cream

TROPICAL OILS
- Palm
- Coconut
- Solid at room temperature

RED MEAT
REFINED SUGAR
- Reserve for special occasions
- Replace sweeteners with natural alternatives (honey, cane syrup)

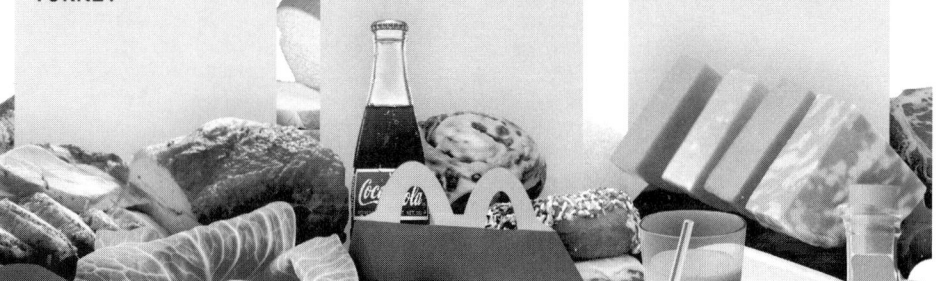

For the Love of Living

Chapter Four

MAKING IT WORK

So, how do you put these principles into practice? Use these guides to help you plan your meals.

One of the reasons we eat in such unhealthy ways is out of convenience, so planning ahead and stocking your pantry with nutritious foods is key to making better choices.

MEAL PLANNING

Make copies of the Weekly Meal Plan to map out your meals for the week and jot down any groceries you need to pick up. On the bottom corner, there is a checklist to help make sure you get your daily recommendations of each food group. Once you've done this for a while, you will get the feel of balanced eating.

1. Try to include a whole grain, healthy fat, and a healthful pro-

tein at each meal, putting plants at the center of the plate and building flavor without excess sugar and salt. Aim for a variety of foods and colors.

2. Total up your day's nutrients to equal ½ vegetables and fruits (about 1/3 veg and 1/8 fruit), ¼ healthy carb (Try to aim for at least half of the grains that you consume to be whole grains) and ¼ healthy protein (fish twice a week).

3. Use healthy fats when cooking, on salad, and in food choices; aim to get less than 10% from saturated fats.

4. Aim to get the daily recommendation of water & liquids (9 cups of water for women, 13 for men).

5. Get the weekly recommendation of exercise (2-1/2 hours of moderate activity per week with strength training for adults).

PANTRY STAPLES GROCERY LIST
You won't always have time to make a meal plan, so having a pantry stocked with nutritious ingredients will set you up for success. Use a pantry staples grocery list to keep your fridge and pantry stocked with a few staples from each food group.

SHOULD I BUY ORGANIC?

According to Harvard Health, although organic foods are growing in popularity and are clearly healthier for the planet, the evidence that they are healthier for people is much weaker. This is due, in part, to insufficient research on the nutrient content of organically grown foods. One widely publicized study from Stanford University found very little difference between the nutritional content of organic and conventional foods, although it did note the pesticide residues were 30% lower on organic produce. However, the British Journal of Nutrition analyzed 343 studies and concluded that organic produce did, in fact, come out on top with 6% higher levels

Making It Work

WEEKLY MEAL PLAN
WEEK OF: _____

SUNDAY
- B
- L
- D

MONDAY
- B
- L
- D

TUESDAY
- B
- L
- D

WEDNESDAY
- B
- L
- D

THURSDAY
- B
- L
- D

FRIDAY
- B
- L
- D

SATURDAY
- B
- L
- D

GROCERY LIST

Dairy

Produce

Grains

Meats

Frozen

Misc.

of vitamin C, 17% higher total antioxidant level, and 25% more of certain phytochemicals. On the downside, the protein content was lower. The benefits of organic foods also include improved flavor and less greenhouse gas emission.

With these benefits comes a higher price as well. In light of this, we have provided some information to help you spend your dollar wisely.

Note that the best way to ensure your produce is organic is to raise it yourself, which can be fun and rewarding!

Dirty Dozen - Foods that have the highest levels of pesticide residues. Most valuable organic produce choices:

1. Apples
2. Celery
3. Cherry Tomatoes
4. Cucumbers
5. Grapes
6. Nectarines
7. Peaches
8. Potatoes
9. Snap peas (imported)
10. Spinach
11. Strawberries
12. Sweet Bell Peppers

If you can, it is also a good idea to buy meat and dairy organically to limit antibiotics and added hormones used in animals.

Note that a more nutritious diet prefers more produce, organic or not, over more meat and dairy.

Clean Fifteen - Foods that have the lowest levels of pesticide residues. Least valuable organic produce choices:

1. Asparagus
2. Avocados
3. Cabbage
4. Cantaloupe
5. Cauliflower
6. Eggplant
7. Grapefruit
8. Kiwi
9. Mangoes
10. Onions
11. Papayas
12. Pineapples
13. Sweet Corn
14. Sweet Peas (frozen)
15. Sweet Potatoes

INCORPORATING MORE FRUITS & VEGETABLES

Incorporating more vegetables and fruits into your diet may seem like a difficult task, but it doesn't have to be! Here are some ways to get started:

VEGETABLES

Slip some in at breakfast - Add vegetables to your omelet or breakfast casserole, a slice of tomato to your egg sandwich, or fajita vegetables to a breakfast burrito.

Add soup as a first course - Vegetable-rich soups (without cream base) like French onion, celery, or pureed carrot soup are a great way to get vegetables in before your main dish, and also aid in eating less during the meal.

Choose vegetables at snack time – Pair hummus, nut butter, or yogurt with bell peppers, carrots, and celery for a nutritious snack.

Prepare vegetables the Mediterranean way – Place any fresh vegetable – carrots, greens, broccoli, cauliflower – in a skillet or sauté pan with a drizzle of olive oil and water. Season as desired and sauté only until crisp-tender for a delicious side dish.

Pair a salad with your main dish (at dinner too) – Fill your bowl with dark green leafy lettuce and toss in your favorite veggies. As a bonus, eating a salad before the main course will help you to consume fewer calories. Avoid creamy dressings to keep salad calories low. A simple dressing can be made with one part olive oil and one part vinegar or lemon juice, seasoned to taste with herbs and pepper.

Roast Vegetables with Baked Dishes - Baking vegetables at 375 degrees F converts the starches to sugar, which releases the deep, nutty sweetness. Drizzle with a healthy oil and bake for 20-25 minutes or until lightly browned. Bake separately or add to casseroles or other dishes. Any vegetable is a great roasting candidate.

Puree vegetables in dishes – Cook and puree vegetables of all sorts like sweet potatoes, carrots, cauliflower, onions, and celery and add to soups, curries, sauces, spreads, and toppings.

FRUIT
Make fruit the star of dessert – Top yogurt with fruit and drizzle with honey, make a frozen fruit yogurt, or try fruit and coconut water popsicles. Bonus: Replacing more sugary desserts with the natural sweetness of fruit will help you keep your calories down. For those special occasions when you want to indulge, you can also include fruit in fruit crisps, pies, bars, and tarts.

Include fruit with breakfast – slicing it on top of hot cereal or yogurt, or eating it along with your breakfast is a great way to get in your daily servings of fruit.

Whip up a smoothie - Puree your fruit for a delicious smoothie for breakfast, or have a small one as a side for lunch or dessert. Skip the extras when wanting to keep the calories down.

Choose fruits at snack time – Fruits are pre-packaged and ready to take if you need something on the go or when you're at home; they are a delicious snack and a great way to get your fruit for the day.

Keep dried fruit in purse or vehicle – When you're hungry and want to grab something immediately, it's a good idea to be prepared. Pack dried fruit in your purse or car for these moments.

HOW TO BUILD FLAVOR NATURALLY
- WITHOUT EXCESS SUGAR, FAT & SALT -

MARINATE
Mix spices and herbs with fresh citrus juice, vinegar, or wine. Coat food thoroughly and refrigerate for an hour before cooking.

ADD CREAMINESS WITH PUREES
- Unsweetened applesauce, pumpkin purée, or squash purée can substitute for oil, eggs, or sugar in some recipes for baked goods.
- Soaked and puréed cashews add richness to soups and sauces.
- Pureed cauliflower replaces potatoes in many recipes.
- Pureed vegetables substitute as a milk base in sauces, soups, and curries.

STEAM-FRY
Get your pan sizzling hot before adding chopped onions and other vegetables. When they begin to stick, stir in a splash of water or reduced-sodium broth.

BALANCE IT ALL WITH BRIGHTNESS

Instead of adding salt to elevate flavors, finish with:
- A splash of vinegar
- A squeeze of citrus juice
- A handful of chopped herbs

ENGAGE THE SENSES WITH HERBS & SPICES

- Garlic adds rich, savory flavor
- Aromatic herbs help build your flavor foundation
- Chiles and chili powder stimulate the palate
- Cinnamon heightens sweet flavors

NATURAL FLAVOR ENHANCERS

Savory
- Stocks and broths
- Fresh or dried herbs
- Wines
- Vinegars
- Ginger, garlic, and onions

Spicy
- Dried and fresh chili peppers
- Mustard
- Curry
- Spices like cumin, turmeric, cardamom, and coriander
- Peppercorns
- Horseradish and wasabi

Sweet
- Fresh and dried fruits
- Fruit juice
- 100% fruit pastes, single strength concentrates, and purees (like applesauce)
- Coconut water

SMARTER SNACKING

It's important to realize that many well-known snack foods are highly processed and packed with more calories and sugar than you bargained for. These foods include muffins (a bran muffin can be loaded with butter and sugar), cereal bars, and energy bars. Other deceitful choices include some fruit leathers, yogurt raisins, and organic candies that often have added sugar and calories.

When choosing snacks, use the same guidelines used for meals – choose whole foods (minimally processed) and focus on plants.

Here are some suggestions:

- 8 oz. plain Greek yogurt with fresh or frozen berries and a sprinkle of granola
- 1 cup raw or herb-roasted nuts or seeds
- ½ cup of low-fat cottage cheese or ricotta and vegetables for dipping
- Handful of grapes with a slice of hard cheese (Cheddar, Swiss)
- 1½ oz. trail mix with dried fruit, dark chocolate, and walnuts
- ¼ cup hummus with 1 cup fresh vegetables
- 1 slice whole-grain bread with 1 tbsp. nut butter and 1 tsp. fruit spread
- 1 banana, sliced and spread with 1 tbsp. nut butter
- 1 cup of popcorn with dusting of dark chocolate shavings

SNACKING STRATEGIES

1. **Don't skip meals** – It's tempting to skip meals to cut calories or when busy but it leads to bingeing later, on snack foods that are usually less nutritious.

2. **Keep junk food out of the house** – One of the best ways to reduce your cravings is to remove junk food from the house where it won't tempt you, and replace it with healthy choices

like a variety of fresh fruits and vegetables. Cutting up your produce and having it ready to go can make it an easier choice as well.

3. **Snack mindfully** – Try not to snack at the kitchen counter or eat out of the bag or box. Portion out your food onto a bowl or plate and sit down to consciously enjoy it. This will help your mind to register when you are full and will cause you to feel more satisfied, as opposed to mindlessly eating a whole bag of chips while reading a book.

4. **Remember, you can take it with you** – Think ahead, and carry a small bag of healthful snacks in your purse or vehicle. If you have a healthy snack handy - preferably, one you really enjoy - you won't turn in desperation to the calorie-laden cookies at the coffee counter or the candy bars in the office vending machine.

5. **Zero in on your hunger** – Often we mistake thirst or boredom for hunger. Drink an 8-ounce glass of water and wait 15 minutes. If you're still hungry, eat a nutritious snack. If you feel unsettled about something, instead of snacking, ask yourself what is bothering you. Jot down your thoughts or take a short walk to help you process your thoughts.

6. **Know your cravings** – It's important to recognize those times when it is appropriate to satisfy your cravings. If you're longing for chocolate, it may be better to actually have a small portion and savor it than snacking on substitutes, which can lead to consuming more calories than what you were craving.

NUTRITIOUS RECIPES
FOR YOU & YOUR FAMILY

Breakfast

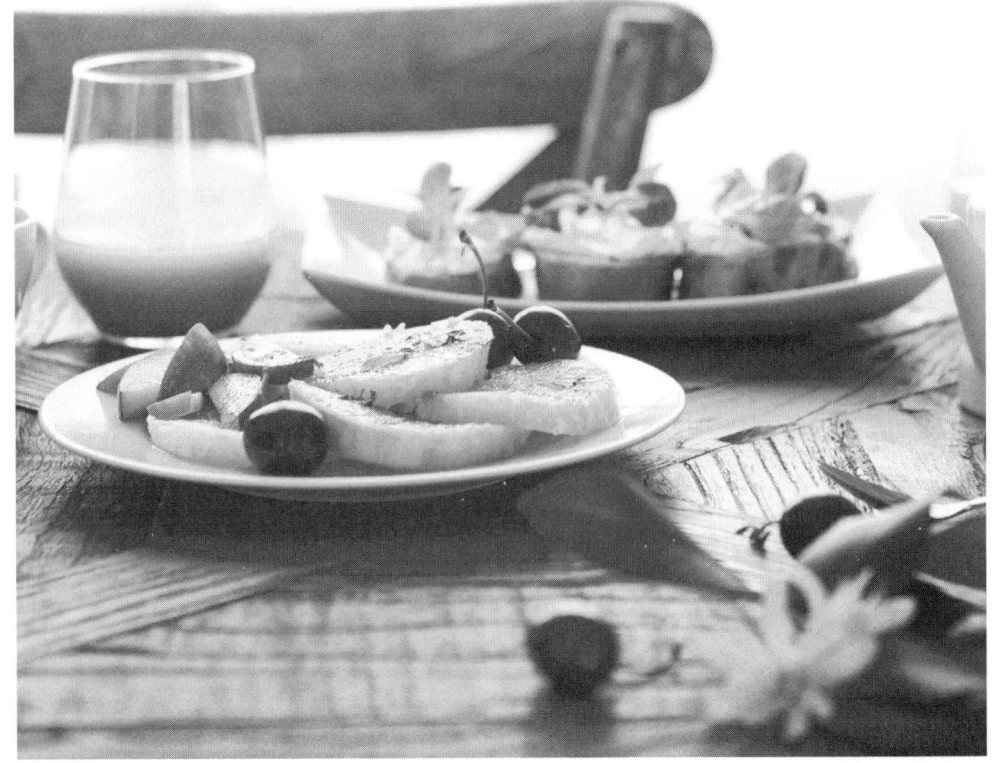

WHOLE-GRAIN PANCAKES

Ingredients

- 1½ cups freshly milled whole grain flour (soft white wheat works well)
- ½ cup all-purpose flour
- 1½ cups sour milk (1½ tbsp. vinegar mixed with 1½ cups milk, allow to sit 3 min)
- ¼ cup sugar
- 1 heaping tsp. baking powder
- 1 tsp. baking soda
- ¼ cup olive oil
- ¼ tsp. salt
- ½ tsp. cinnamon
- 1 egg, separated

Combine the dry. Add the wet and the egg yolk, keeping the egg white aside, stir the batter until smooth. Whisk the egg white until foamy and fold into the batter. Measure out pancakes using a ¼ cup measure or ladle. Cook pancakes on a hot griddle or in a hot frying pan until bubbles pop, turn once and cook until golden.

* Add 1-1½ cups fresh or frozen blueberries to the batter to create delicious blueberry pancakes.

* Topping options - use 1½ cups fresh or thawed blueberries, strawberries, or peaches. Crush and add a small amount of honey or sugar. Pour over your pancakes along with real maple syrup.

ALMOND BUTTER BANANA OATMEAL SMOOTHIE

Ingredients

- ½ cup steel cut oats or rolled oats
- 1 cup Silk almond milk
- 1 tbsp. almond butter
- 1 tbsp. honey
- 1 whole banana
- 1 handful ice

Combine all but ice in blender and puree. Add ice.

QUICK AND EASY GRANOLA

Ingredients

- 8 cups rolled oats
  (rolling your own is best, but you can also use steel cut, quick oats, or purchased rolled oats)
- ½ cup wheat germ
- ½ cup oat bran
- 3 tbsp. whole flax seed
- ¾ cup sliced almonds
- ½ cup chopped pecans
- ¾ cup shredded coconut
- Butter
- Honey
- Vanilla
- Cranberries or raisins

Mix this all together and set aside. In a saucepan over medium heat, melt 2 sticks of butter and add 1 cup honey. Remove from heat and add 1 tsp. vanilla and a ½ tsp. cinnamon. Stir and pour over the dry mix. Stir to coat completely. Spread onto 2 jellyroll pans and bake at 350 degrees for 12 minutes. Stir and then bake for another 12-15 minutes until golden brown. Remove and cool completely. You may wish to add 1 cup dried cranberries or raisins before placing in an airtight container for storage.

APPLE-BERRY SMOOTHIE

Ingredients

- ½ cup blueberries
- ½ apple, chopped
- 1/3 cup Greek yogurt
- 8 almonds
- 1 tbsp. honey
- 1 cup (almond) milk

In a blender, combine the berries, apple, yogurt, almonds, honey, and milk until smooth.

3 INGREDIENT PANCAKES

by: Natalie Jill, sports nutritionist

Ingredients

- 1 egg, beaten
- 1 banana (ripe is preferred), mashed
- 1 tbsp. almond butter (or other nut butter)
- 1 tbsp. coconut oil
- ½ tsp. vanilla extract
- Cinnamon to taste

Heat coconut oil in a pan at medium/low heat. Mix egg, banana, and almond butter to create your batter. You can add vanilla extract and/or cinnamon. Pour batter into pan in pancake dollops (if batter is thin, add a little coconut flour). Once bubbles pop open, the pancakes are ready to be flipped.

OPTIONAL BERRY TOPPING

Ingredients

- 1/3 cup fresh or frozen berries
- 1 tsp. coconut oil
- Zest of ½ lemon

Heat coconut oil in a saucepan. Add berries and lemon zest and cook until soft. Top pancakes with berry topping and enjoy.

BREAKFAST CASSEROLE

Ingredients

- 20 oz. potatoes, peeled & cut into ½ inch cubes
- 1 lb. turkey sausage
- 1 onion, diced
- 1 red pepper, diced
- 3 garlic cloves, minced
- 2 cups shredded cheddar cheese
- 6 eggs
- ⅓ cup low-fat milk
- ¼ tsp. black pepper
- Sliced green onion

Preheat oven to 375 F. Cook the potato dices in salted boiling water for about 5 minutes. Drain and let cool.

Heat a skillet to medium-high and cook the sausage until browned. Break it up in the process. Remove from skillet with a slotted spoon. Leave 1 tbsp. of grease.

Cook the onion and red pepper in the sausage grease for about 5 minutes. Add the garlic and cook a few more minutes. Place into a large baking dish (9x13 inches) together with sausage and potato dices.

In a bowl, whisk together the eggs, milk, and black pepper and pour into the baking dish. Add 1-1/2 cups of the shredded cheese and stir to combine.

Sprinkle the remaining cheese on top, cover with foil and bake for 20 minutes. Uncover and continue baking for 10-15 more minutes.

Let the breakfast bake rest for a few minutes. Add sliced green onion and serve hot.

Lunch

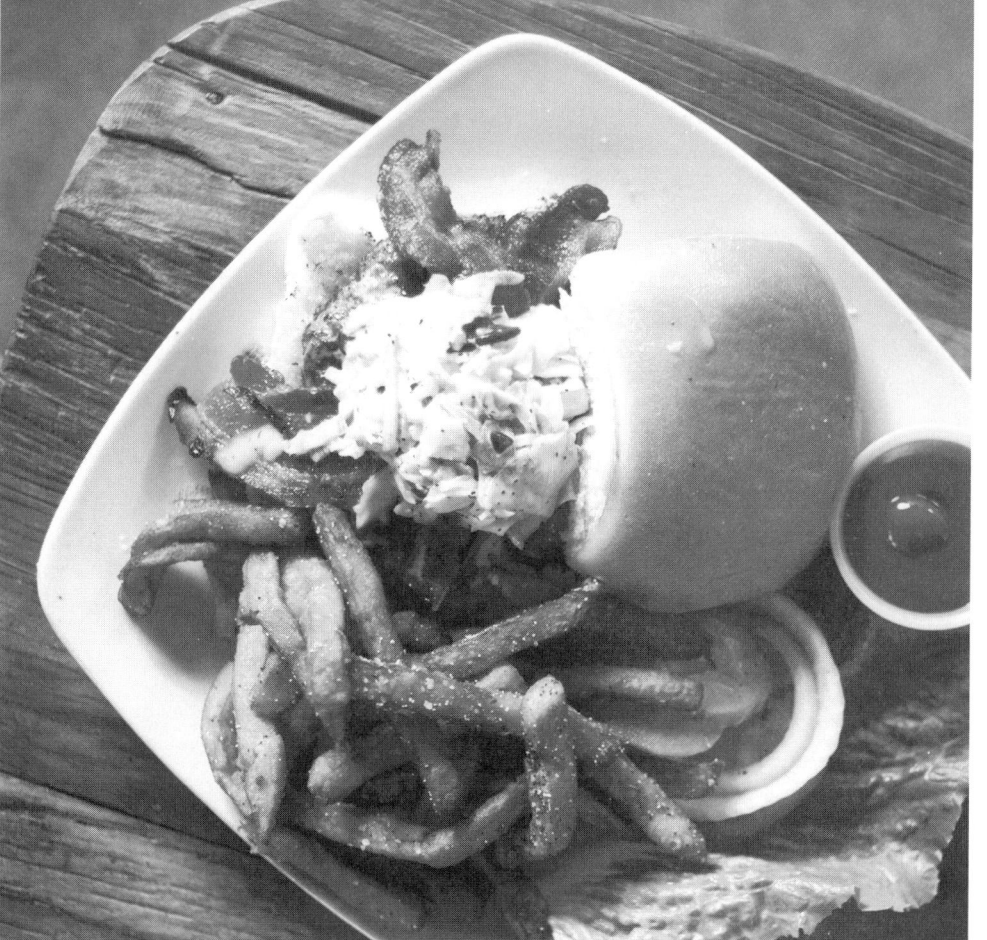

CURRIED TUNA SALAD SANDWICH

SERVES: 2

Ingredients

- 4 oz. can of tuna packed in oil, or 2 hard-boiled eggs
- ½ carrot, diced
- ½ celery stalk, diced
- 2 tbsp. red onion, diced
- 1 tsp. curry powder
- Salt and pepper, to taste
- 2 slices bread
- ½ avocado

Toast bread. Toss tuna (with oil from the can), curry spice, vegetables, salt, and pepper in a bowl (if using eggs add 1-2 tbsp. oil to the mixture; combine and mash the eggs with the other ingredients in the bowl, using a fork). Cut avocado in half and scoop ½ of it out of its skin; spread on toast, using a fork to mash into the bread. Place tuna (or egg) mixture on the avocado. Delicately season with salt and pepper to taste. Serve open face. Wrap the remaining half of the avocado in an airtight plastic bag, with the nut, and store in the fridge.

CHICKEN, BRUSSELS SPROUTS & QUINOA SALAD

Ingredients

- 1 (leftover) lemon-basil chicken breast, chopped into chunks
  Vegetarians: leftover lemon-basil chickpeas
- ½ cup pre-cooked quinoa
- 1½ cups salad leaves
- 1 celery stalk (or approximately 4 pre-cut sticks), chopped into chunks
- Brussels sprouts (leftover)
- 2 tbsp. vinaigrette

Place salad leaves, leftover Brussels sprouts, quinoa, celery, and chicken or chickpeas in a portable lunch container. Store vinaigrette in small container. Keep in a cool place until lunch. When you're ready to eat, toss the ingredients together.

BLACKENED FISH TACOS WITH AVOCADO-CILANTRO SAUCE

SERVES: 6

Ingredients

For the Blackened Fish:
- 1½ lbs. tilapia fillets
- 1½ tsp. smoked paprika
- 1 tsp. garlic powder
- 1 tsp. dried oregano
- 1 tsp. onion powder
- ½ tsp. cumin
- ½ tsp. salt
- ½ tsp. brown sugar
- ¼ tsp. cayenne pepper
- 2 tbsp. canola oil
- 12" corn tortillas

For the Slaw:
- ½ red cabbage, sliced thin
- ¼ green cabbage sliced thin
- ½ medium-sized onion diced
- ½ cup cilantro
- Juice of 1 lime

For the Avocado-Cilantro Sauce:
- ½ cup sour cream
- 1 ripe avocado, pitted and skinned
- ¼ cup cilantro, chopped
- Juice of 1 lime
- 1 jalapeno, chopped and seeded
- Salt, to taste

In a small bowl, combine the smoked paprika, garlic powder, dried oregano, onion powder, cumin, salt, brown sugar, and cayenne pepper. Sprinkle the mixture over both sides of your tilapia fillets, and then rub the seasonings in.

Combine all of the Avocado-Cilantro Sauce ingredients in a food processor or blender. Pulse until well combined.

Combine all of the Slaw ingredients in a large bowl and mix well.

Heat the oil in a heavy-bottomed pan over medium-high heat. Once heated, add in the tilapia (a few at a time if you can't fit them all at once). Cook for 4-5 minutes on each side, or until the outside is blackened and the fish flakes apart easily. Remove the fish from the heat, and if desired, warm the corn tortillas in the same skillet over medium heat, cooking for about 30 seconds on each side. Break up the tilapia into 2-3" pieces. Stack the tortillas in twos. Distribute the fish evenly between the 6 sets of tortillas, and top with Slaw and Avocado-Cilantro Sauce. Serve.

STRAWBERRY AVOCADO SPINACH SALAD WITH CHICKEN

SERVES: 2

Ingredients

- ¼ cup extra virgin olive oil
- 1 tbsp. golden balsamic vinegar
- 1 tsp. lemon juice
- 1 tbsp. fresh tarragon, roughly chopped
- ¼ tsp. kosher salt
- ¼ tsp. freshly ground black pepper
- 2 boneless, skinless chicken breasts
- 6 cups fresh spinach, loosely packed
- 6-8 large strawberries, hulled and quartered
- 1 avocado, peeled, seeded, and cut into chunks
- ¾ red onion, thinly sliced rings
- ¼ cup feta cheese
- 2 tbsp. sliced almonds

Whisk the extra virgin olive oil with the balsamic vinegar, lemon juice, tarragon, kosher salt, and freshly ground black pepper in a small bowl until blended.

Place the chicken breasts in a shallow bowl and cover with half of the dressing, cover and refrigerate for 30 minutes to 2 hours.

Spray a grill pan or 12-inch non-stick pan with cooking spray and heat to medium-high. Place the chicken breasts on the hot grill pan. Cook for 3 minutes then flip the chicken breasts. Cook for another 3 minutes, and turn. Reduce the cooking temperature to medium low and cook the chicken for 20-25 minutes more, turning every 5 minutes or so. Cooking time will depend on the thickness of the chicken, but it will be done when it hits 165 degrees internal temperature. Let the chicken rest for 5 minutes then slice into ¼ inch slices.

Arrange the spinach, strawberries and red onion in a bowl. Lightly toss with the remaining dressing. Add the avocado and sliced chicken and top with feta and almond slices. Serve immediately.

CHOPPED AVACADO, FETA, & BARLEY SALAD

Ingredients

- 1 cup cooked (leftover) barley
- 1½ cups salad leaves
- ½ avocado
- ½ cup cherry tomatoes
- 4 tbsp. feta cheese
- 2 tbsp. vinaigrette

Combine ingredients and enjoy.

CUCUMBER SALMON SALAD

Ingredients

- 1 (leftover) cooked salmon fillet
- 1 ½ cups salad leaves
- ½ avocado
- ½ cucumber, chopped
- Juice of half a lemon
- 1 tbsp. olive oil
- Salt and pepper to taste

Combine ingredients and enjoy.

SIDE SALAD WITH QUINOA

Ingredients

- Cup of salad
- 1 tbsp. vinaigrette
- ½ cup precooked quinoa

Plate a cup of salad. Top with quinoa and a tablespoon of vinaigrette.

Dinner

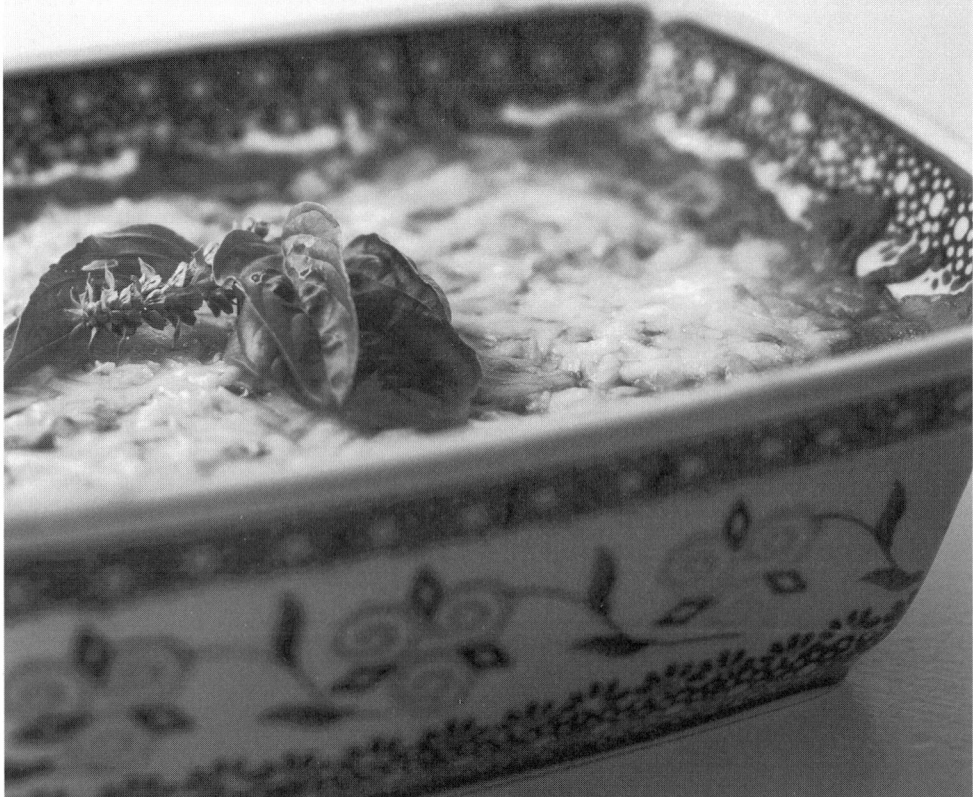

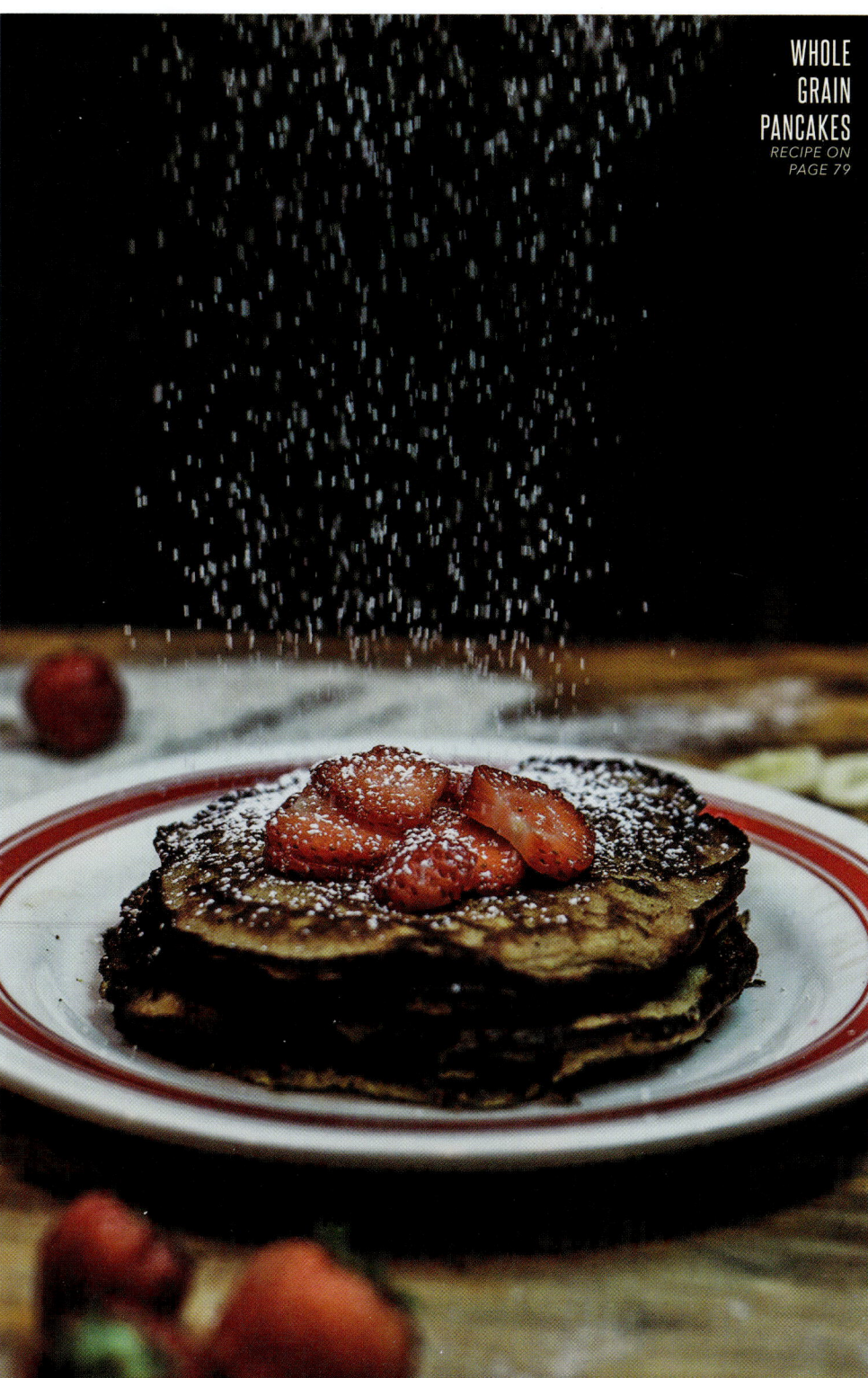

WHOLE GRAIN PANCAKES
RECIPE ON PAGE 79

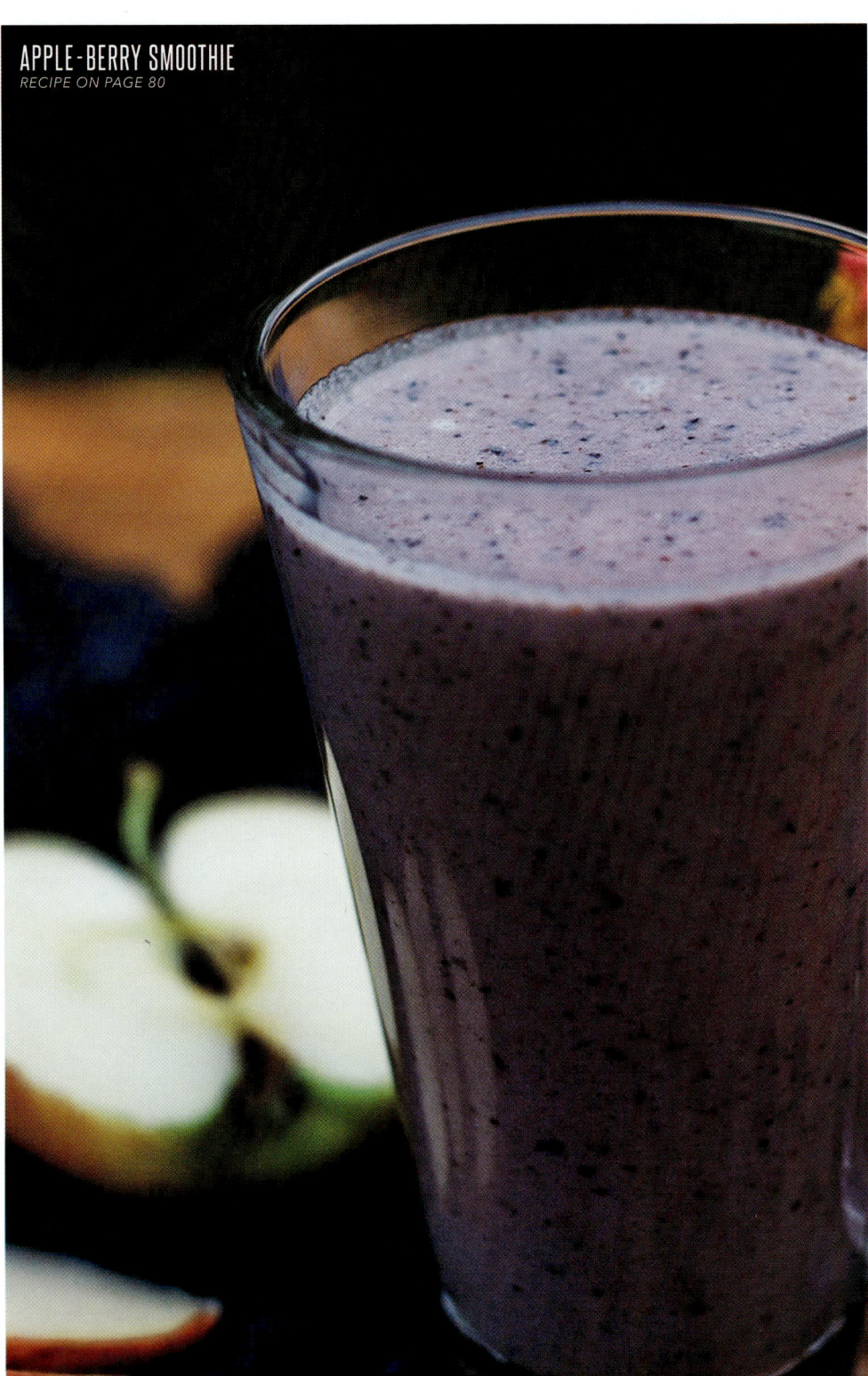

APPLE-BERRY SMOOTHIE
RECIPE ON PAGE 80

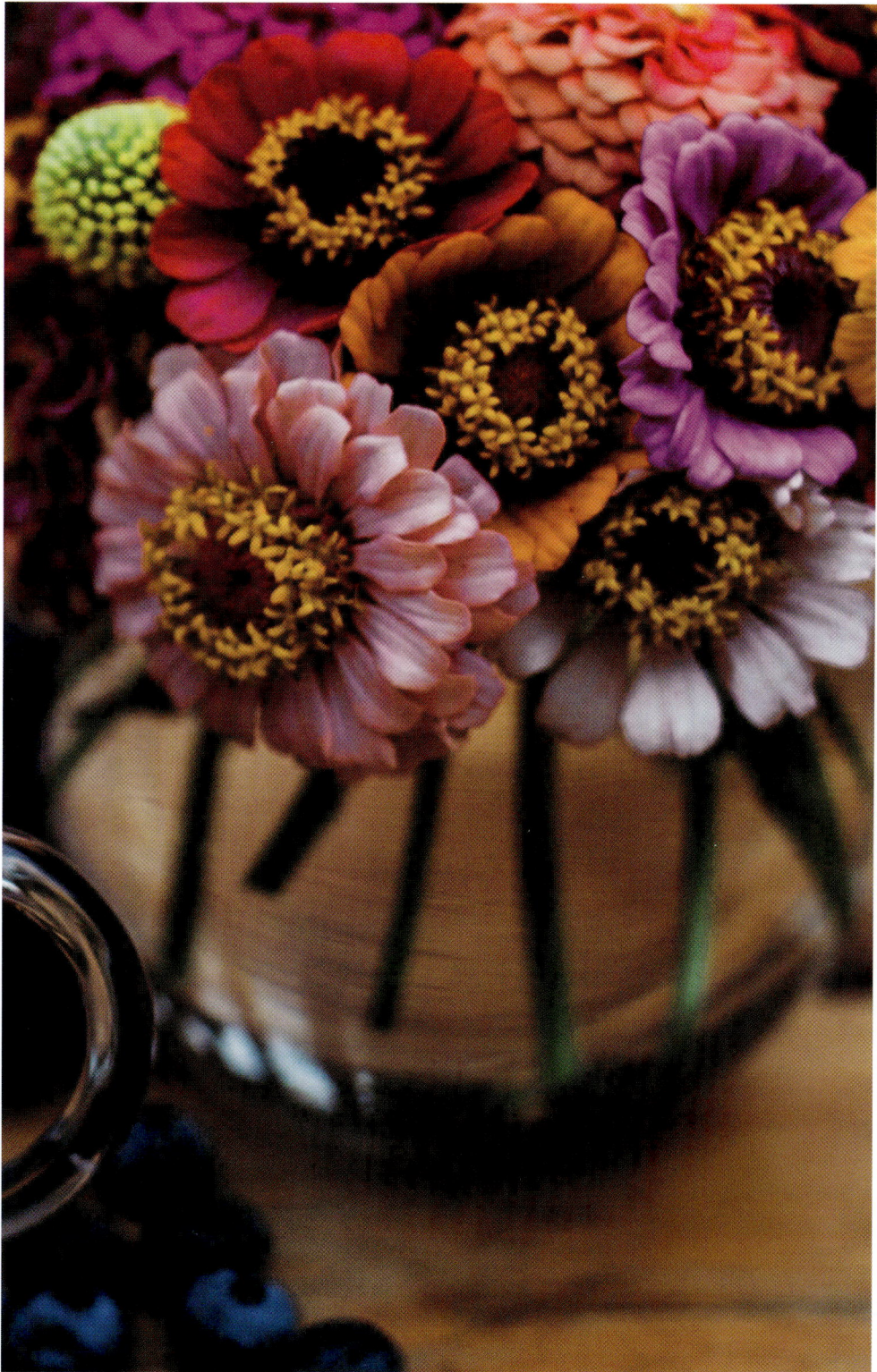

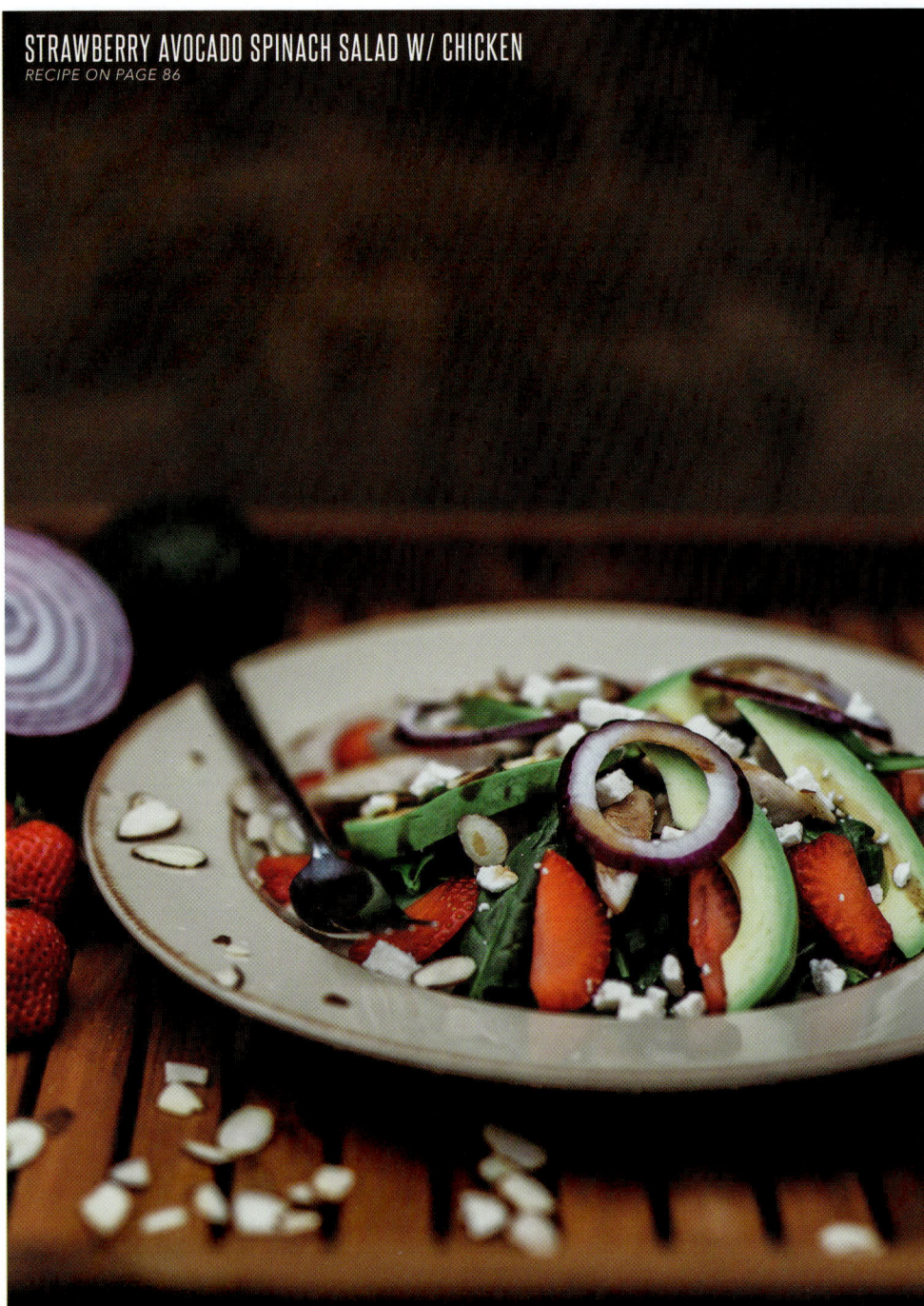

STRAWBERRY AVOCADO SPINACH SALAD W/ CHICKEN
RECIPE ON PAGE 86

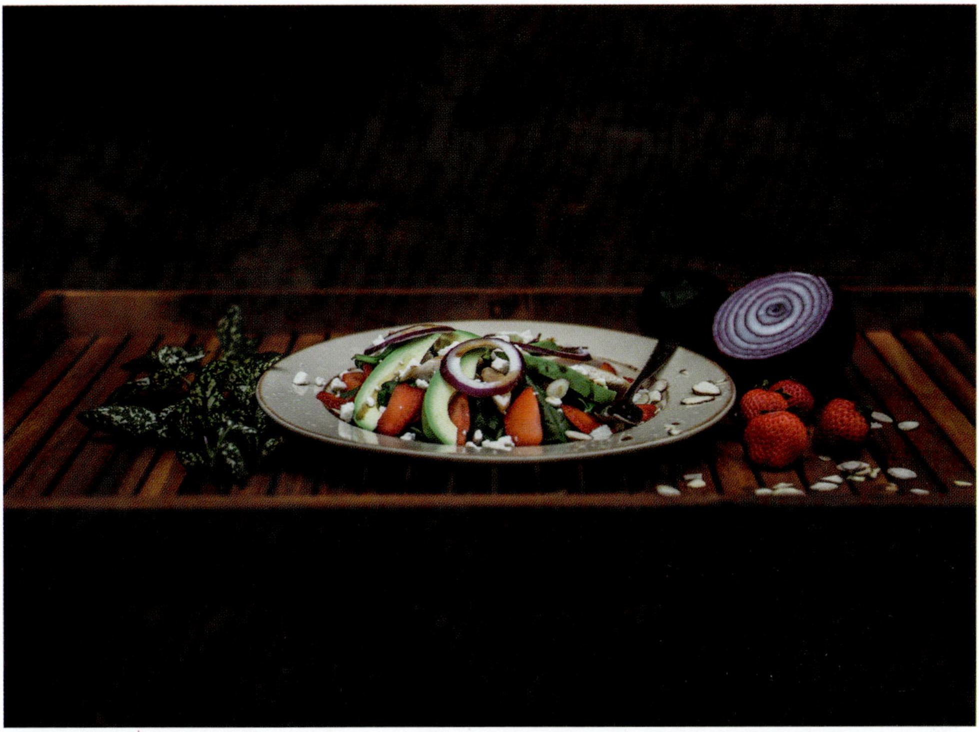

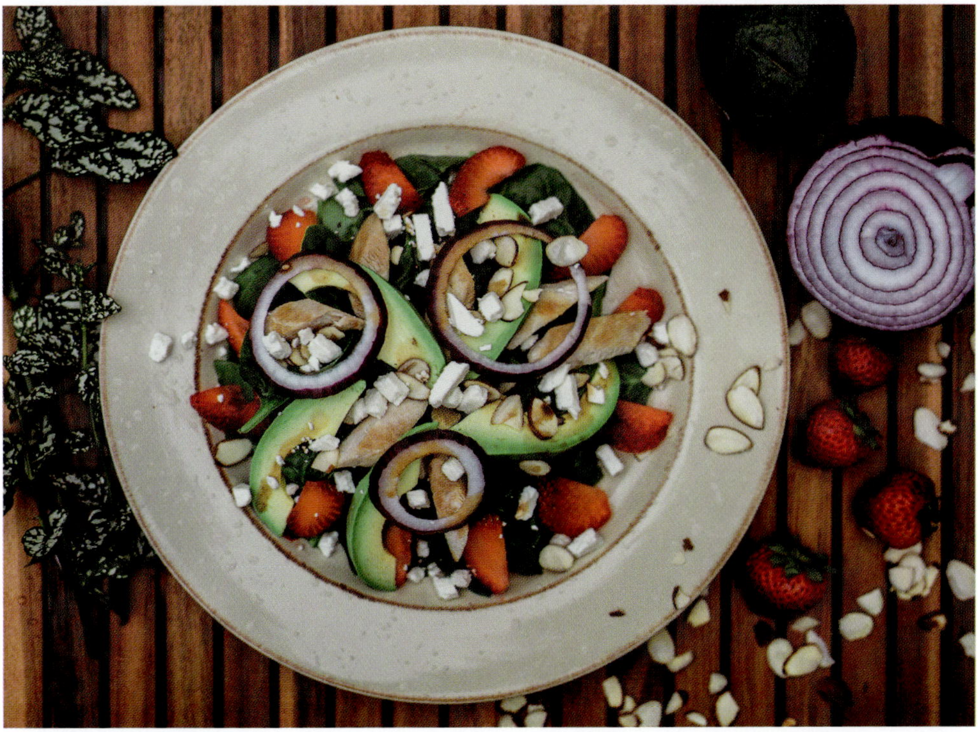

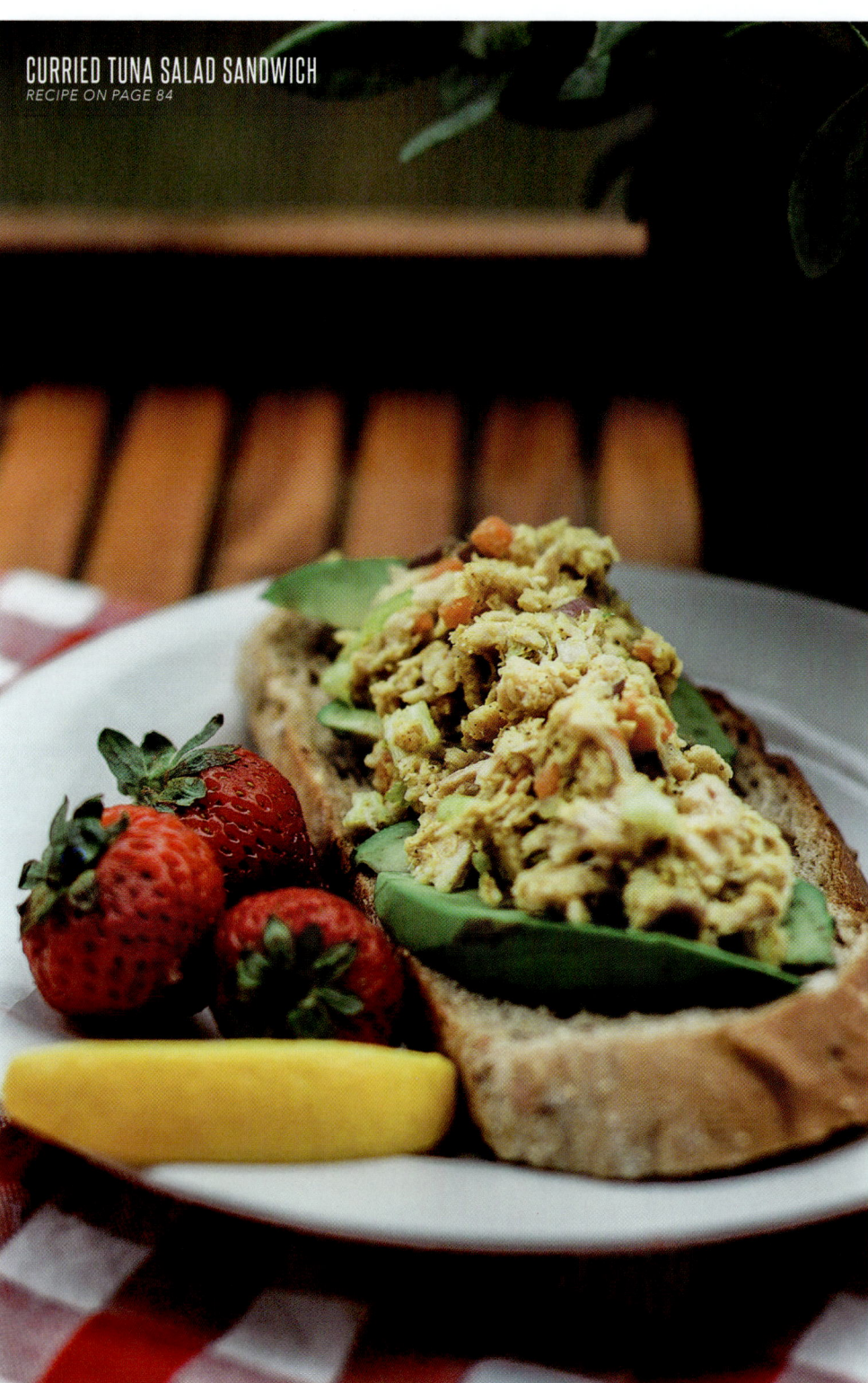

CURRIED TUNA SALAD SANDWICH
RECIPE ON PAGE 84

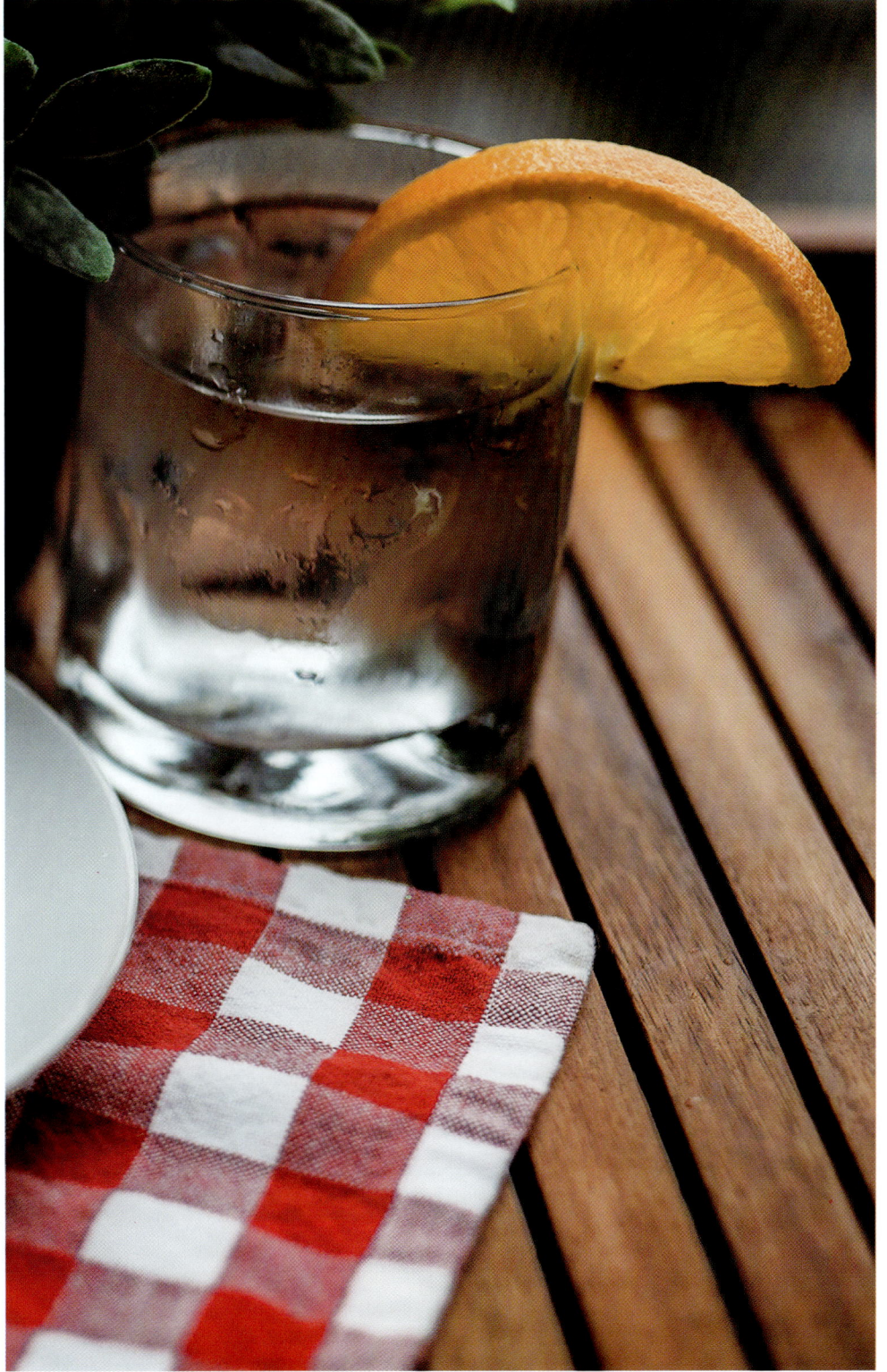

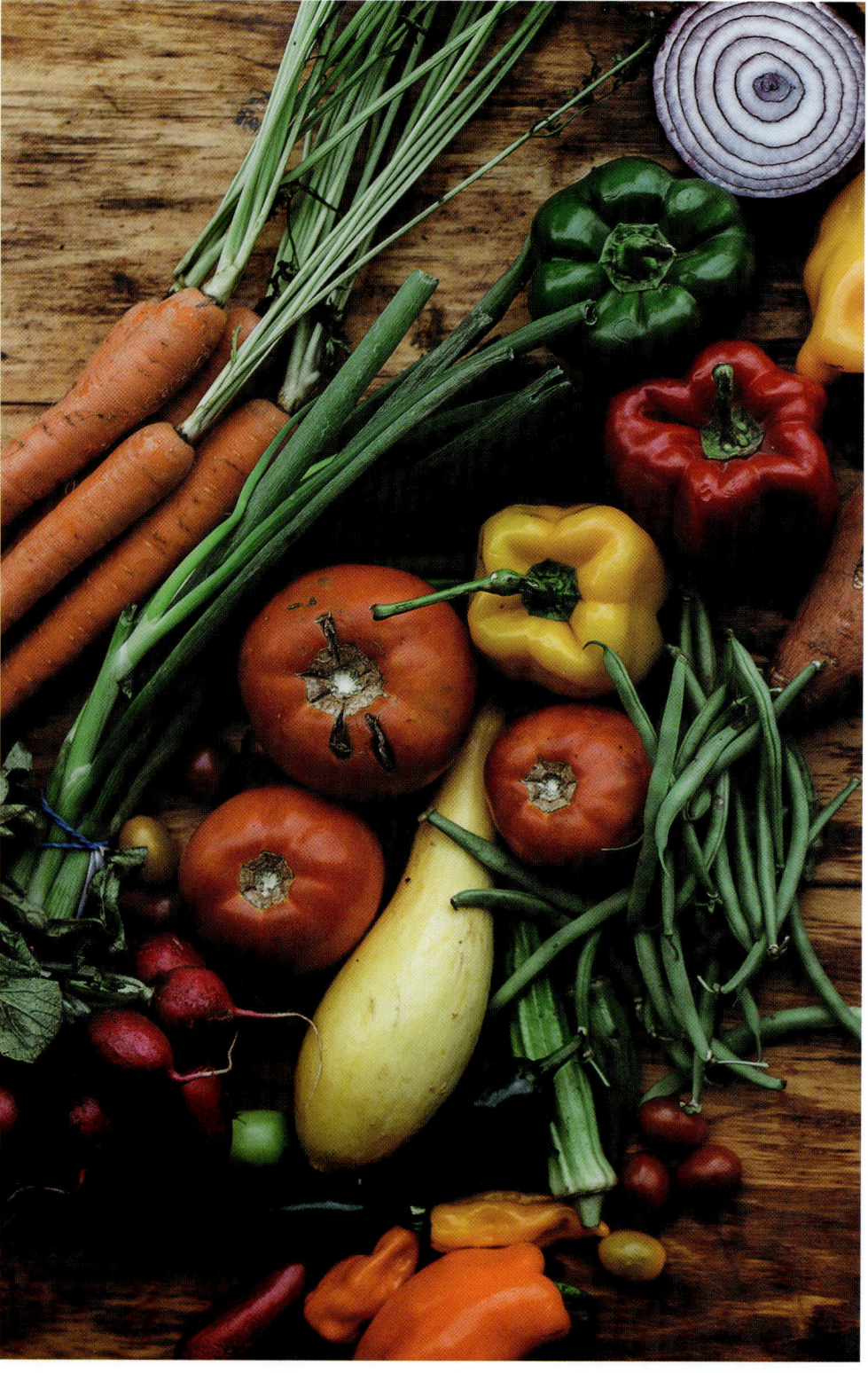

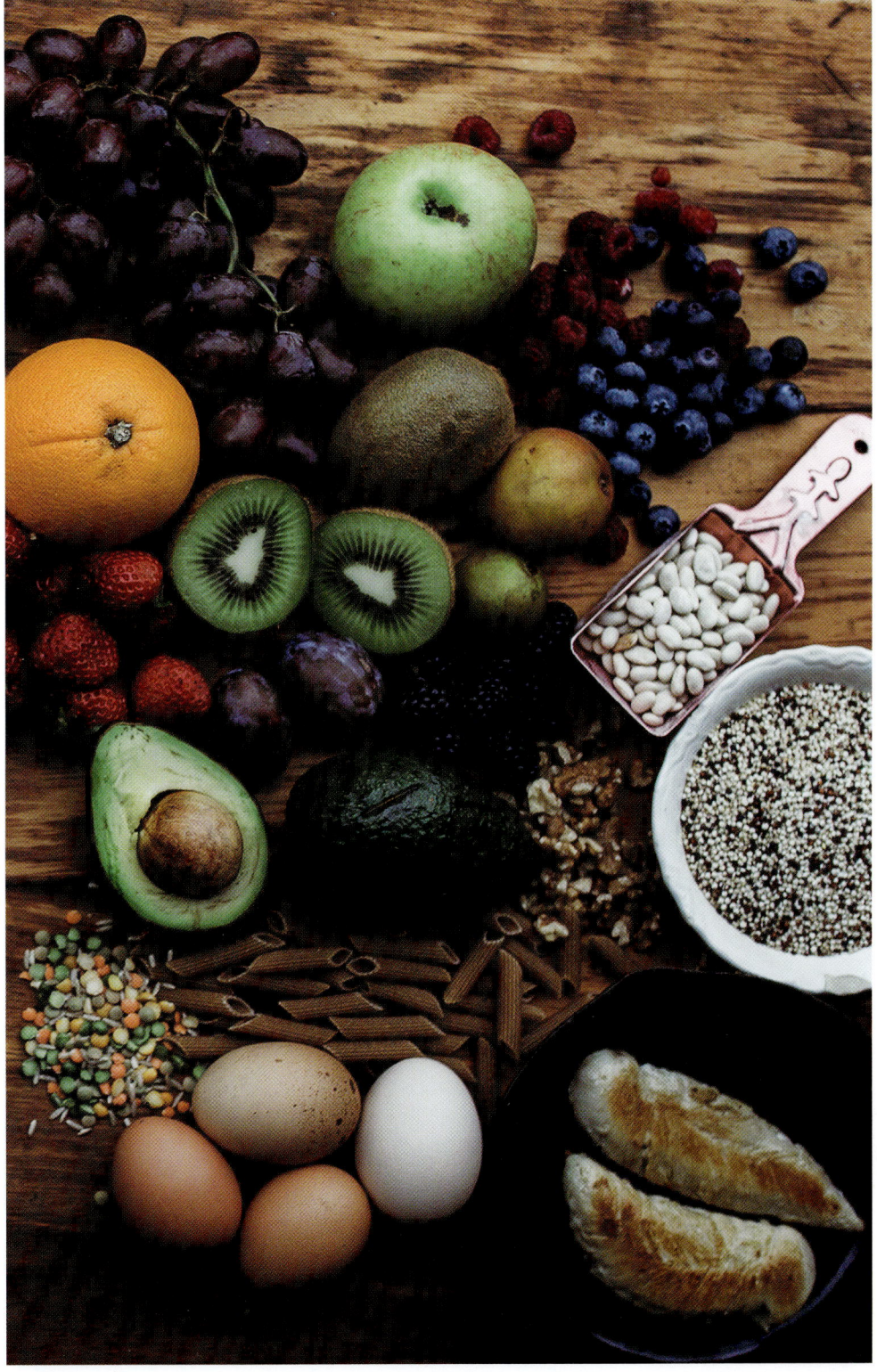

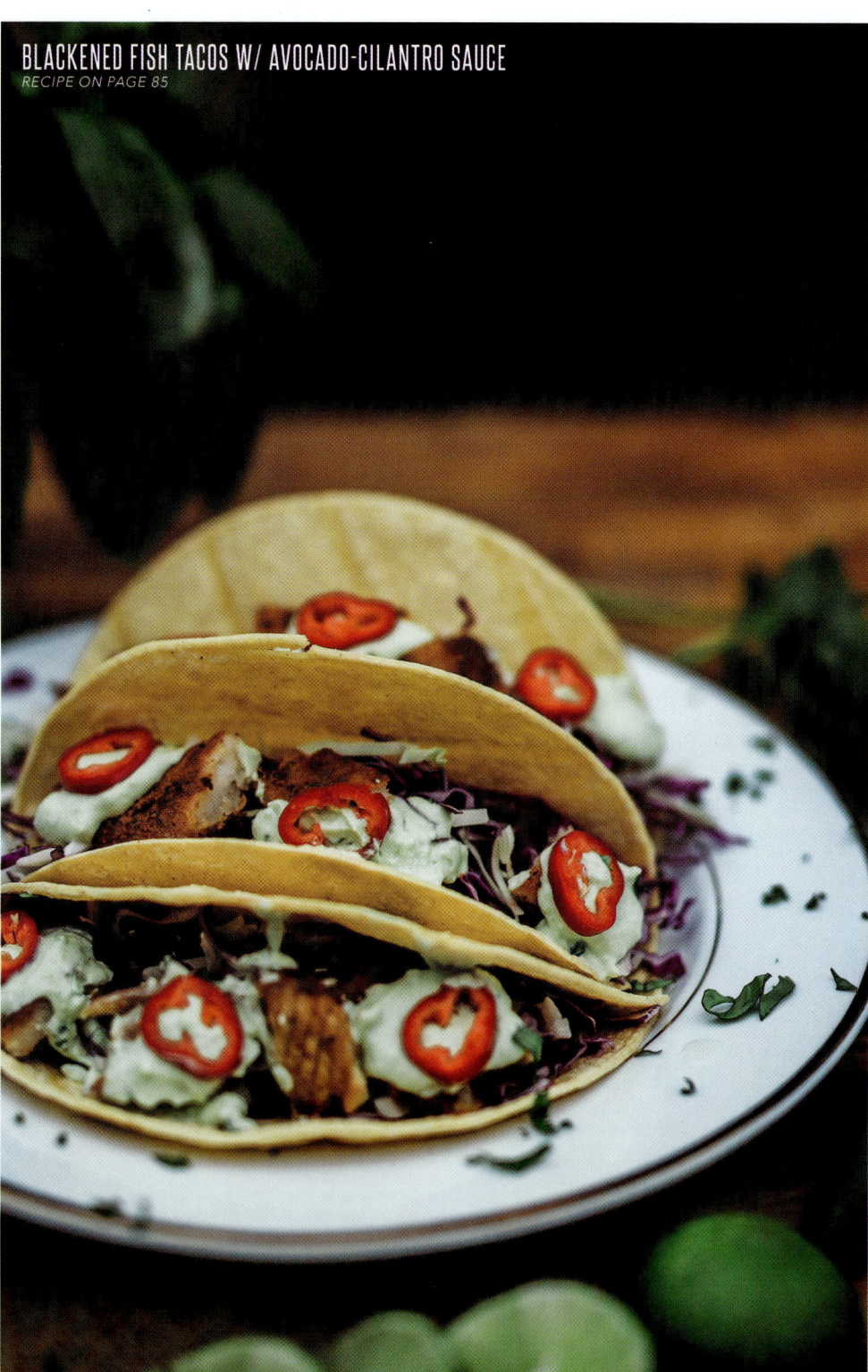

BLACKENED FISH TACOS W/ AVOCADO-CILANTRO SAUCE
RECIPE ON PAGE 85

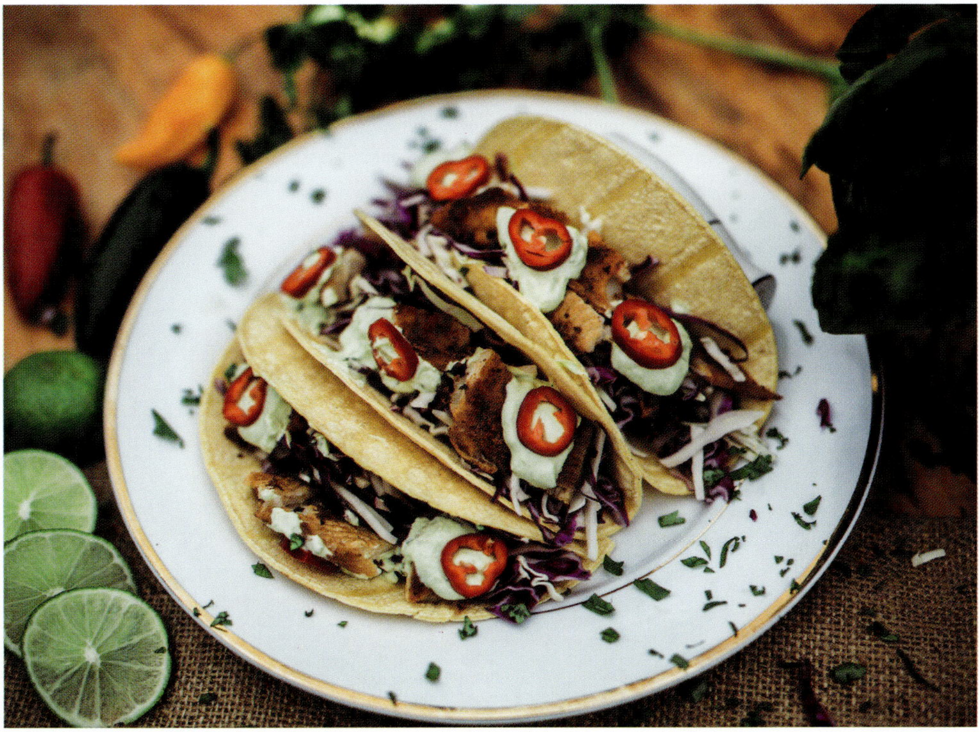

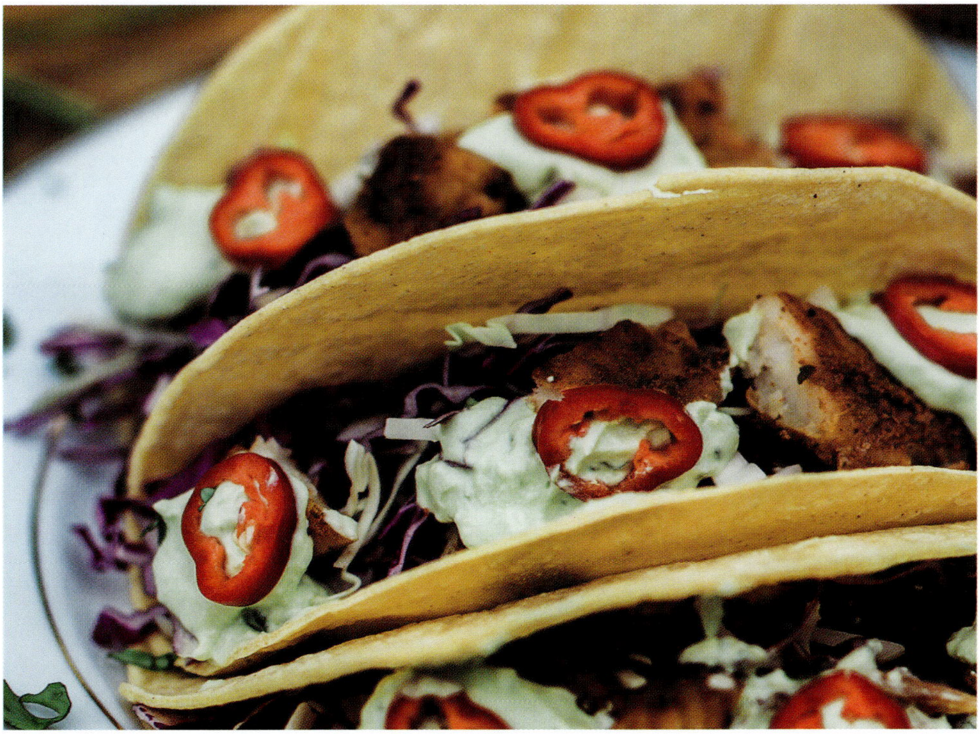

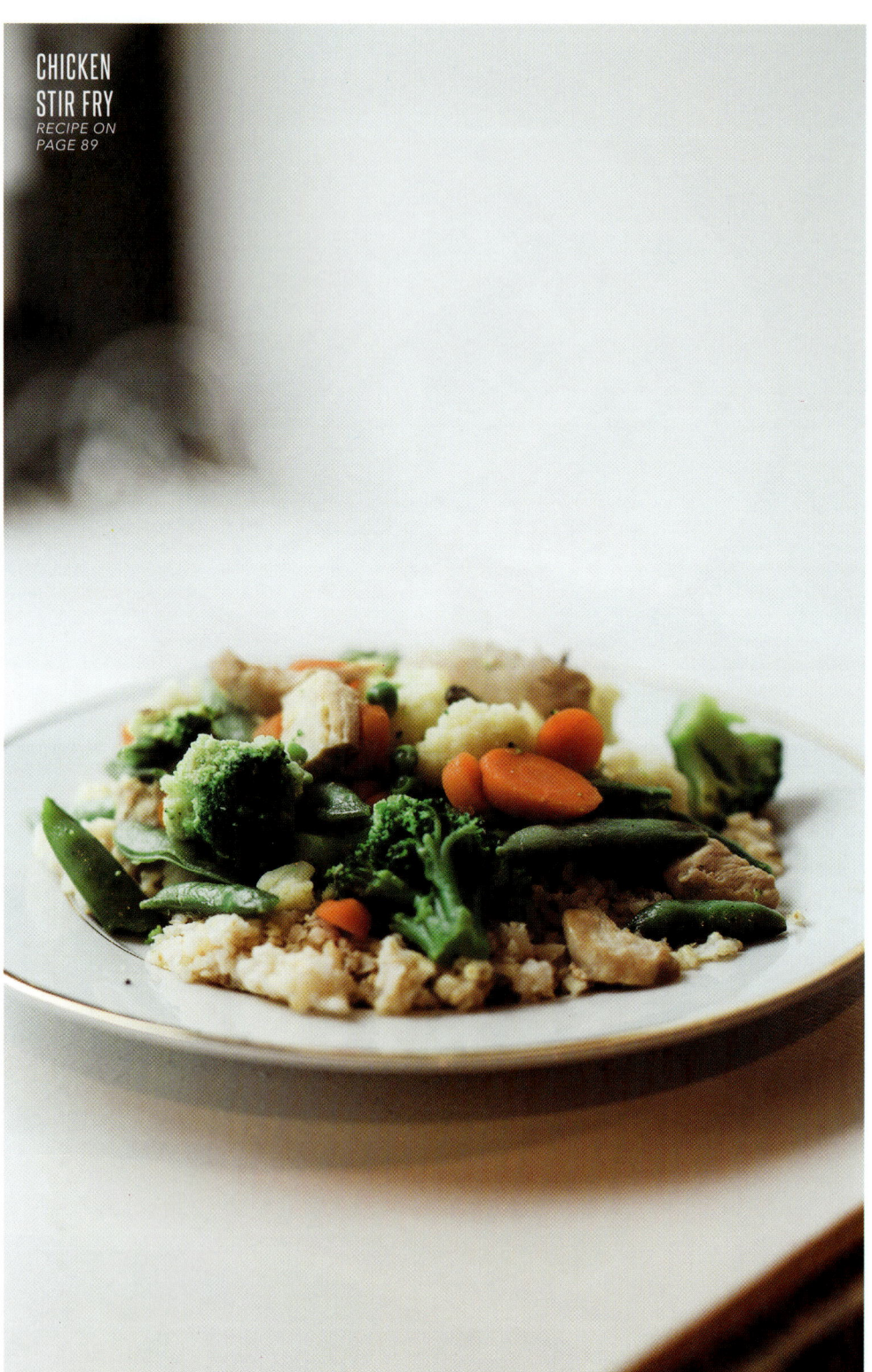

CHICKEN STIR FRY
RECIPE ON PAGE 89

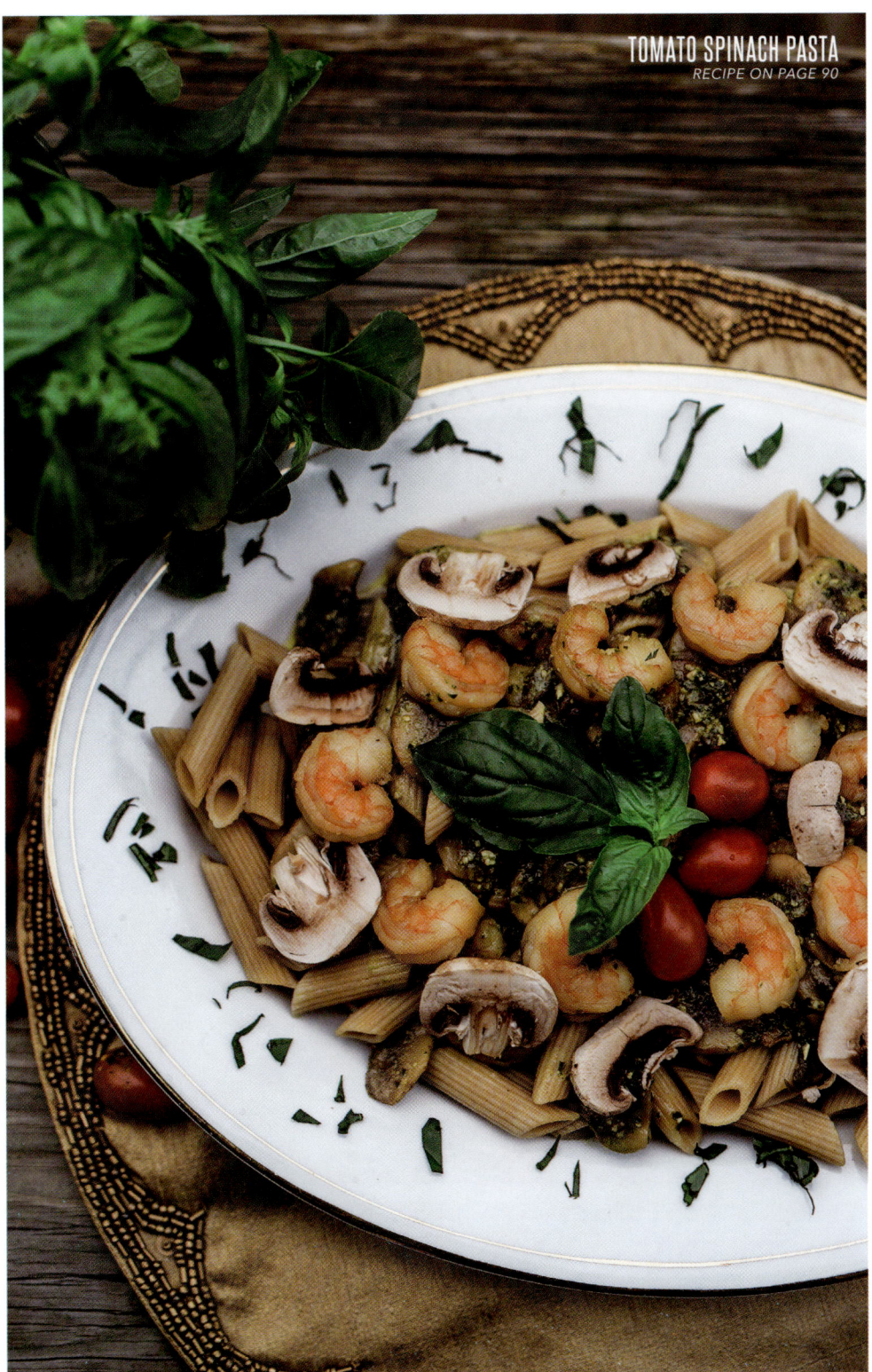

TOMATO SPINACH PASTA
RECIPE ON PAGE 90

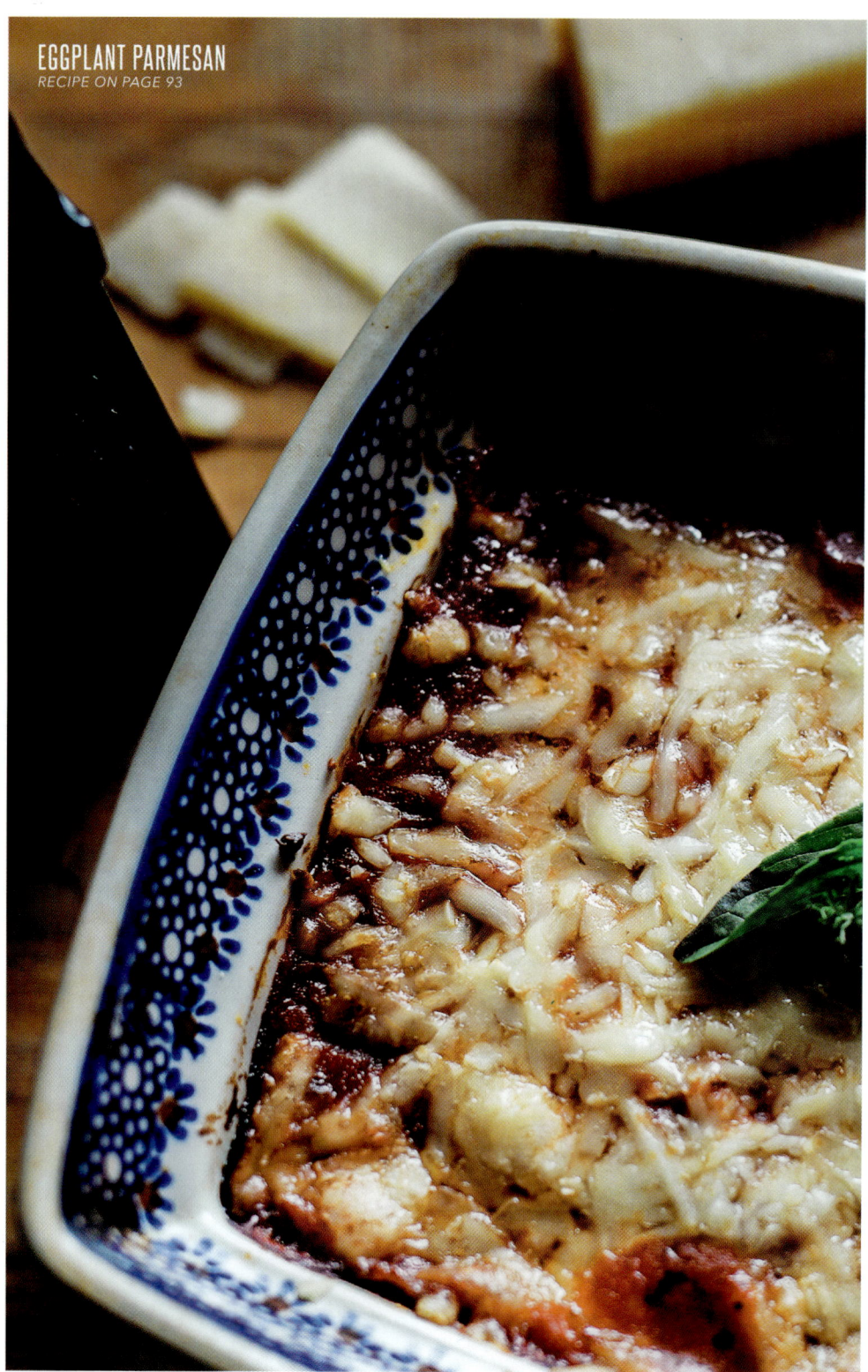

EGGPLANT PARMESAN
RECIPE ON PAGE 93

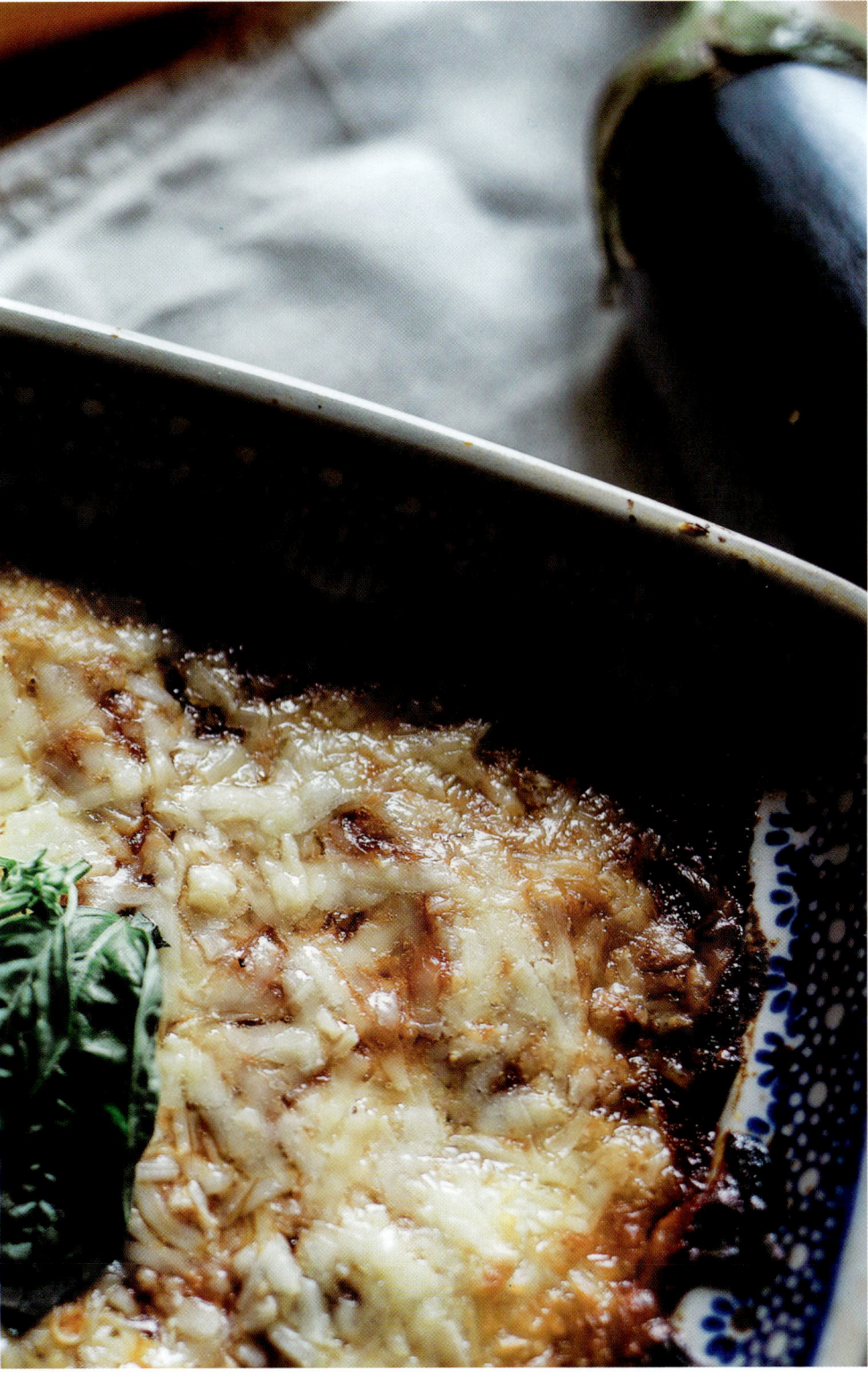

MASHED CAULIFLOWER
RECIPE ON PAGE 92

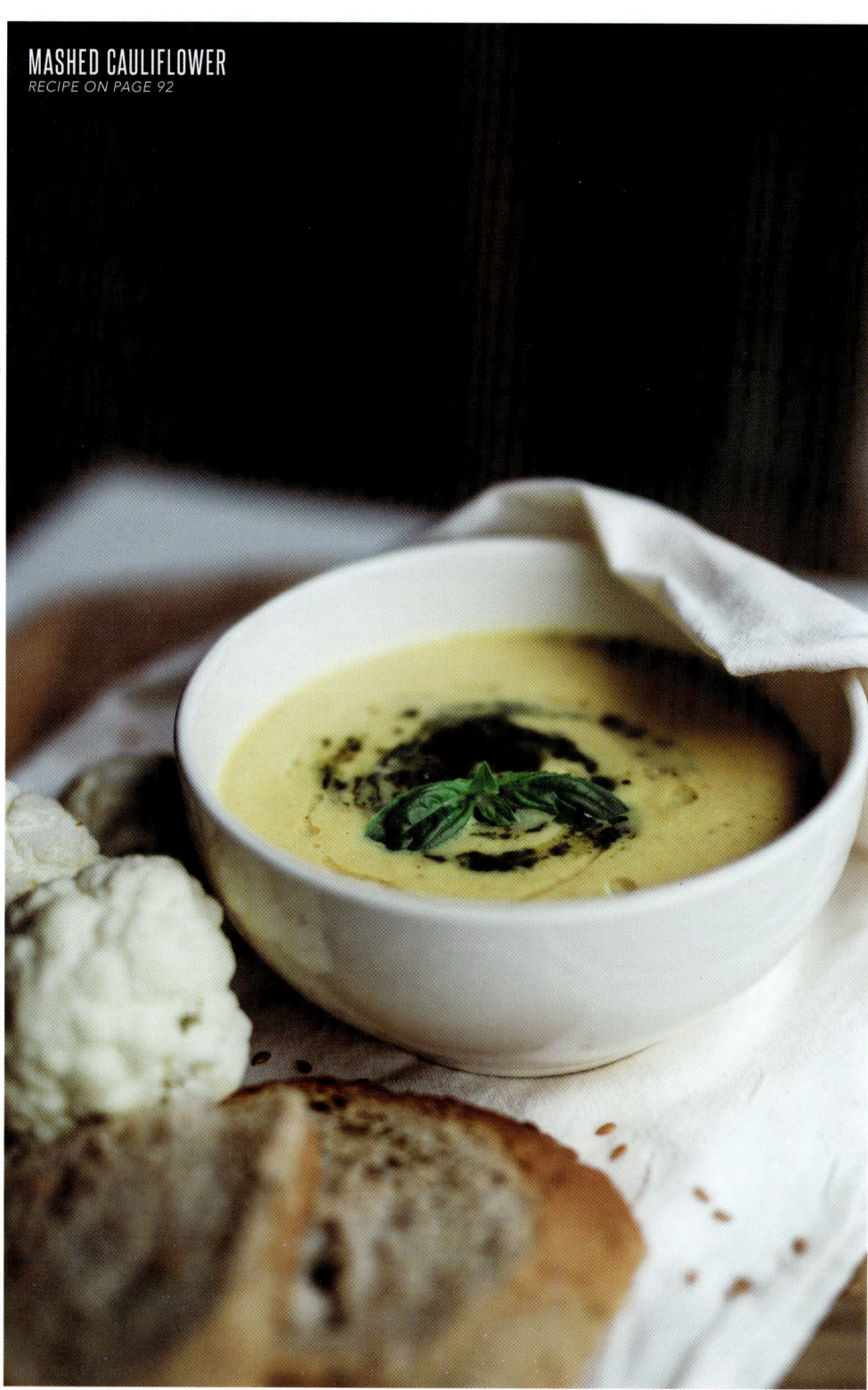

CHICKEN STIR-FRY

Ingredients

- 1-1½ lb. fresh chicken tenders, cut into bite-sized pieces
- Olive oil
- 2 heads of broccoli florets
- 2 cups cauliflower
- 1 cup carrots, chopped
- ½ cup fresh snow peas, optional
- ¼ cup onion, diced
- ½ cup peas
- 1 cup water, warm
- 5 tbsp. soy sauce
- 4 tsp. cornstarch
- 2 tsp. sugar
- ½ tsp. garlic powder
- 4 tsp. beef bouillon

Brown chicken tenders in olive oil, remove and set aside. Sauté vegetables in olive oil until crisp/tender, place with chicken. Combine remaining ingredients in a small bowl, mix and pour over chicken and vegetables. Heat to boiling and reduce to thicken. Serve over rice.

CHICKEN BURGERS

Ingredients

- 2 lb. chicken, ground
- 1 egg, beaten
- ½ cup bread crumbs
- 1 tbsp. seasoned salt
- Olive oil
- 1 cup fresh mushrooms, chopped
- ½ cup onion, diced
- 2 tsp. garlic, minced
- ½ cup carrot, finely chopped
- ¼ cup green pepper, diced

Sauté vegetables in olive oil until tender. Remove and cool. In a large bowl, combine chicken, egg, breadcrumbs, and seasoned salt. Stir in cooled vegetables. Form into patties and grill. Delicious on a whole-wheat bun with lettuce, tomato, bacon, and mayonnaise.

TOMATO SPINACH PASTA

Ingredients

- 1 tbsp. olive oil
- 1 small onion, diced
- 2 cloves garlic, minced
- 1 can diced tomatoes
- ½ tsp. oregano
- ½ tsp. basil
- ½ tsp. salt
- ¼ tsp. pepper
- 2 tbsp. tomato paste
- 2 oz. cream cheese
- 2-3 pieces of bacon, fried and crumbled or diced
- ¼ cup Parmesan cheese, grated
- ½ lb. whole grain penne pasta
- ½ bag spinach

In a large saucepan, bring water to a boil and cook the pasta al dente. Drain and set aside. In a large saucepan, sauté the onion and garlic in olive oil. Add the tomatoes, bacon, and spices. Add tomato paste and ½ cup water. Stir. Turn down the heat, cut in the cream cheese and whisk until smooth. Add the Parmesan and stir once again. Add the spinach and stir 35 minutes to wilt. Add pasta and toss to finish.

BROWN SUGAR BBQ SALMON

Ingredients

Mix the marinade:
- 2 tbsp. brown sugar
- 4 tsp. vinegar
- 4 tsp. honey mustard
- ½ tbsp. soy sauce
- ½ tbsp. lemon juice

Whisk together and pour over the salmon fillets. Marinate 3-4 hours, refrigerated. Grill, skin side down, on medium heat for 10-14 minutes until the fish flakes easily.

BAKED FRENCH FRIES

Ingredients

- 3-4 large potatoes, unpeeled and cut into long wedges
- 1 tsp. olive oil
- Seasoned salt

Preheat the oven to 425 degrees. Coat a baking sheet with nonstick spray. Place the cut potatoes, oil, and seasoned salt in a bowl with a lid. Cover and shake to coat. Pour into the baking pan and bake for 15 minutes. Turn, sprinkle with additional seasoned salt and bake 5 minutes more until potatoes are soft and golden.

VEGGIE COUSCOUS

Ingredients

- 2 medium carrots, diced
- ½ cup celery, chopped
- ¼ cup onion, chopped
- ½ green pepper, julienned
- 1 medium zucchini, diced
- 2 tbsp. olive oil
- ¼ cup minced fresh basil
- ¼ tsp. salt
- 1 ½ cup chicken broth
- 1 cup uncooked couscous

Sauté the vegetables in oil for 4 minutes. Add the basil, couscous, salt, and broth. Bring to a boil, cover, remove from heat and let stand 8 minutes. Fluff with a fork and serve.

CHICKEN BURRITOS

Ingredients

- 1 tbsp. olive oil
- 1 ½ cup chicken, cooked
- 1 can pinto or black beans, drained and rinsed
- ½ cup fresh salsa
- 1 can green chilies
- ¾ cup water
- Adobo seasoning
- 1 can green chilies
- 1 tsp. lime juice
- ¼ tsp. salt
- ¼ cup fresh cilantro, chopped
- Tortillas
- White rice, cooked
- Monterey jack cheese

Heat olive oil in a saucepan. Add salsa, water, adobo seasoning, green chilies, beans, and lime juice; stir together. Add chicken, salt, and cilantro. Stir and cook for 2 minutes. Warm tortillas and add some cooked white rice, chicken mixture, grated Monterey jack cheese, and salsa into each one. Roll tightly closed, and grill until the tortilla is crispy on each side. Serve with chopped lettuce, tomato, salsa, and sour cream or guacamole.

MASHED CAULIFLOWER

SERVES: 4

by: Natalie Jill, sports nutritionist

Ingredients

- 1 head cauliflower
- 4 tbsp. butter
- ½ tsp. salt
- ½ tsp. ground black pepper
- 1-2 cloves garlic

Chop the cauliflower into 2-inch pieces. Steam the cauliflower and garlic until tender. Place the cauliflower and garlic in a food processor or blender; add the butter, salt, and pepper. You may add any other spices you like. Puree until smooth.

EGGPLANT PARMESAN

Ingredients

- 1 large eggplant, ¼" slices
- 2 eggs
- 3 tbsp. water
- ⅓ cup seasoned breadcrumbs
- ⅛ tsp. salt
- Olive oil
- 2 cups marinara sauce
- 2 cups mozzarella cheese, shredded
- ⅓ cup Parmesan cheese, grated

Preheat oven to 375 degrees. Beat eggs and add water, whisk. Add salt to the breadcrumbs and stir. Dip each slice of eggplant into the egg mix and then the breadcrumbs. In a large skillet over medium heat, fry the eggplant slices until golden.

Spread some sauce in the bottom of a 13x9 pan. Place one-half of the eggplant slices into the pan; follow with half of the sauce and cheeses than repeat the layers, finishing with the cheeses on top. Bake until heated through, and the sauce is bubbly.

HEALTHY YUMMASETTI

Ingredients

- 1 lb. grass-fed ground beef
- 1 - 8 oz. bag of medium noodles
- Condensed tomato soup substitute (see recipe)
- Basic cream sauce w/ celery (see recipe)
- Sliced cheese
- Parsley

Brown 1 lb grass-fed ground beef. Drain. Cook 1 - 8 oz, bag of medium noodles. Drain. Mix one batch of condensed tomato soup substitute (see recipe). Mix one batch of basic cream sauce with celery (see recipe). Combine all together and place in a greased casserole dish. Top with sliced cheese and sprinkle with parsley. Bake at 350 degrees for 30 minutes or until heated through and cheese begins to brown.

EGGPLANT LASAGNA

SERVES: 6
by: Natalie Jill, sports nutritionist

Ingredients

- 2 tbsp. extra virgin olive oil
- 1 small onion
- 4 cloves garlic
- 1 lb. ground turkey or beef
- 1 – 28 oz. can crushed tomatoes
- 1 – 6 oz. can tomato paste
- Salt and pepper to taste
- 1 tbsp. fresh parsley, chopped
- 1 tbsp. fresh basil, chopped
- ¼ cup Parmesan cheese
- 1 large egg
- 16 oz. cottage cheese (can substitute with ricotta)
- 1 lb. fresh spinach
- 8 oz. mozzarella cheese, grated
- 1 large eggplant
  (sliced thin, lightly sprinkle with salt and press moisture out with a towel)
- Parchment paper
- Tin foil

Preheat oven to 400 degrees. Heat 1 tbsp. oil in skillet over medium heat, add onion and cook for 2 minutes. Add garlic and cook for another minute. Add ground turkey or beef and cook about 10 minutes. Once turkey is fully cooked, add tomatoes, tomato paste, salt, and pepper and simmer for 20 minutes. Beat the egg in a medium bowl, then stir in cottage cheese, ½ cup parmesan cheese, salt, and pepper and set aside.

In a separate skillet, add 1 tbsp. oil and cook spinach over medium heat until wilted.

Spread 1/3 of meat sauce in bottom of a 9x13 baking dish. Layer with 1/2 of sliced eggplant.

Sprinkle on 1/3 of the mozzarella cheese, 1/3 of the cottage cheese mixture and ½ of the spinach. Repeat the same layering process starting with the meat sauce. After the spinach layer, finish with the last 1/3 of meat sauce and remaining mozzarella and parmesan cheese.

Line a piece of tin foil with parchment paper, then coat parchment paper with olive oil. Cover lasagna, parchment side down. Cook for 20 minutes or until bubbly. Let stand for 5 minutes before serving.

VEGETABLE PIZZA

by: Natalie Jill, sports nutritionist

Ingredients

- 1 spaghetti squash, roasted
- 1 lb. Italian turkey sausage or regular sausage
  (Nitrate free, natural, seasoned the way you like)
- 3 eggs, whipped
- 1 zucchini, chopped
- ½ brown onion, chopped
- 1 orange pepper, chopped
- 12 oz. mushrooms, chopped
- 1 cup pizza sauce
- 1 tbsp. olive oil
- 1 avocado, sliced

Preheat oven to 400 degrees. Cut spaghetti squash in half lengthwise, add a little salt and pepper and olive oil and bake face down for about 30-45 minutes. Heat olive oil in pan and cook onions until soft and clear. Add meat and sauté until cooked. Add veggies and cook until soft. Preheat oven to 400 degrees. Line an 8x8 dish with spaghetti squash. Add mixture of meat and vegetables. Pour in pizza sauce and mix well. Finally, add whipped egg and mix well. Cook for 45-60 minutes. Allow to cool, and serve with sliced avocado.

SWEET POTATO FRIES

by: Natalie Jill, sports nutritionist

Ingredients

- 4 sweet potatoes, peeled and sliced into ¼ inch strips
- 2 tbsp. olive oil or coconut oil
- Cinnamon or pumpkin pie spice (optional)

Pre-heat oven to 400 degrees. Cut sweet potatoes; it is okay to make them any size you want; be sure they aren't too thick, or they will take longer to cook. In a sealed bag, put in potatoes, add olive oil. Shake bag until fries are evenly coated with oil. Place fries on prepared baking sheet and bake until tender, depending on size, about 40 minutes. Sprinkle with cinnamon or pumpkin pie spice (optional).

HEALTHY FRIED RICE

SERVES: **1**
by: Natalie Jill, sports nutritionist

Ingredients

- ½ cup brown rice (already cooked)
- 4 egg whites, scrambled
- Braggs Aminos, sprinkle to taste

Combine and enjoy.

VEGETABLE BEAN FAJITAS

SERVES: **4**

Ingredients

- 2 tsp. extra-virgin olive oil
- 1 large onion, sliced
- 1 green bell pepper, sliced
- 1 red bell pepper, sliced
- 2 small zucchinis, sliced
- 4 oz. fresh mushrooms, sliced
- 2 cloves garlic, minced
- ¼ jalapeno pepper, finely diced
- 1 tbsp. fresh lemon juice
- 1 tsp. cumin
- 1 tsp. chili powder
- ¼ cup cilantro, chopped
- 2 cups unsalted cooked beans (e.g. pinto, red)
- 8 small corn tortillas
- 1 cup guacamole (make your own with mashed avocado, lemon juice, and garlic)
- 1 cup salsa (look for lower sodium brands if not homemade)

Heat olive oil in a large skillet (cast iron works best). Add onion, bell pepper, zucchini, mushrooms, garlic, and jalapeno and sauté for about 10 minutes, until just tender. Add lemon juice, cumin, chili powder, and stir well. Sprinkle with chopped cilantro.

To serve: Fill tortilla shells with beans and vegetable mixture and garnish with guacamole and salsa.

LEMON BASIL BUTTER CHICKEN

SERVES: 2

Ingredients

- 1 tbsp. olive oil
- ½ tbsp. butter
- 2-4 oz. chicken breasts
- Juice of half a lemon
- 6 torn basil leaves
- Salt and pepper, to taste

Heat oil and butter in a frying pan over low heat. When melted, turn heat to medium and add chicken to the pan. Cook on medium, approximately 5 to 7 minutes per side. When the breasts turn to white, add lemon juice and basil. Cook for another minute or two. Season to taste with salt and pepper. Plate the chicken breast you wish to eat and top with some juices from the pan. Conserve the other in the fridge for tomorrow's lunch.

TOMATO AND WHITE BEAN SOUP

Ingredients

- 4 tbsp. olive oil
- 1 medium onion, chopped
- 2 celery stalks, chopped
- 3 carrots, chopped
- 1 - 14 oz. can of diced tomatoes in juice
- 1 can of white beans
- 1 - 17 oz. box of vegetable broth
- 4 tbsp. fresh basil, chopped
- Salt and pepper, to taste
- Parmesan cheese

In a large pot, heat oil over medium heat. Add the onions and cook until they are translucent, stirring occasionally. Add celery and carrots to the pot, and cook over medium heat until they are soft, about 5 to 7 minutes. Add the beans, vegetable broth, and tomatoes with their juice, and bring to a boil. Lower heat to a simmer, add basil, and allow the mixture to reduce, stirring occasionally. Simmer for about 40 minutes. When it's ready, ladle a portion into a bowl and sprinkle with parmesan cheese. Pack up the rest for tomorrow's lunch.

SESAME-ROASTED TURNIPS WITH BARLEY

Ingredients
Barley
- ½ cup uncooked barley
- 1-1½ cups water

Sesame Roasted Turnips
- 1 large turnip
- 1 clove garlic, minced
- 1 tbsp. olive oil
- 2 tsp. sesame seeds
- 2 tsp. honey
- ¼ tsp. salt
- 1 tbsp. soy sauce
- 1 cup cooked barley

Note: Get the barley boiling first, then put the turnips in the oven.

Barley: Follow the cooking instructions on the package or combine water and barley in a small pot on the stove and bring to a boil. Cover and reduce heat to low until the barley has absorbed the liquid, about 30 minutes. Plate half the barley (about one cup) and store the other half in the fridge for tomorrow's lunch.

Turnips: Preheat oven to 375 degrees. Cut turnips into ¼ inch cubes and place in a bowl. Add minced garlic, olive oil, sesame seeds, honey, and salt: toss until well combined. Spread turnips into a single layer in a roasting pan and bake for 25 to 30 minutes until caramelized and tender. Remove from oven and add the soy sauce. Serve over cooked barley.

SOY SALMON WITH STIR-FRIED QUINOA

Ingredients

Soy Salmon
- 2 - 6 oz. salmon fillets
- 2 tbsp. olive oil
- 2 tbsp. soy sauce
- Juice of half a lemon and grated zest
- Salt and pepper, to taste

Stir-Fried Quinoa
- 2 tbsp. olive oil
- ½ red onion, chopped
- ½ carrot, finely chopped
- ½ celery, finely chopped
- ½ cup pre-cooked quinoa
- 2 tbsp. sesame seeds
- Salt and pepper, to taste

Note: Begin preparing the vegetables while the oven is heating. It'll only take a moment to get the fish ready and by the time it's cooked, your vegetables will be done.

Soy Salmon: Preheat oven to 400 degrees. Line a baking sheet with foil or parchment paper. Place salmon on the baking sheet. Sprinkle with olive oil, lemon juice, and lemon zest; season with salt and pepper. When the oven is ready, cook the salmon for about 10 minutes or until it's opaque. Remove the salmon from the oven, sprinkle with soy sauce, and return to the oven for another 2 minutes. Plate one fillet, and conserve the other for tomorrow's lunch.

Stir-Fried Quinoa: In a frying pan, heat oil over medium for about 1 minute and then add the onions. Cook until they are translucent. Add the celery and carrots and cook until soft, about 7 minutes. Stir in the quinoa and sesame seeds and heat for about 2 minutes. Season with salt and pepper. Plate the quinoa and enjoy with the salmon.

SPINACH & FETA PIE WITH CHICKPEA FLOUR CRUST

SERVES: 6

Ingredients

- 1 cup chickpea flour
- 1 tbsp. olive oil
- ¾ tsp. salt
- 1 cup water
- 1 lb. frozen spinach, thawed, moisture squeezed out
- 2 eggs
- ¾ cup feta cheese, crumbled
- ½ cup low-fat cottage cheese
- ¼ tsp. salt
- Black pepper

Note: If you can't find chickpea flour you can substitute another flour or bake the filling without a crust, in a greased cast-iron skillet.

Preheat oven to 500 degrees. Use cooking spray to lightly mist a cast-iron skillet; place skillet in oven and heat for at least 10 minutes. In a large mixing bowl, whisk together crust ingredients; chickpea flour, olive oil, salt, and water, until there are no lumps. Remove hot skillet from the oven. Pour batter for crust into skillet. Return to oven for 10 minutes. In a separate bowl, combine spinach with eggs, feta, cottage cheese, and salt. Mix well. Remove skillet from oven, and reduce oven temperature to 400 degrees. Spread spinach filling evenly over crust, sprinkle with black pepper, and bake for 20 minutes. Cool for 10 minutes before slicing into six pieces.

BROILED SHRIMP WITH LEMON

Ingredients

- Shrimp
- Lemon
- Salt

Peel the shrimp and, with a sharp knife, make a shallow cut along the back and remove the vein. Sprinkle with lemon juice and a small amount of salt. Place the shrimp under the broiler about 3 inches from the heat. Broil 3 minutes, turn and broil three minutes more. Do not overcook - shrimp should be cooked just until the flesh is opaque. Serve with more lemon juice if desired.

SIMPLE CHICKEN CURRY

Ingredients

- 2 tbsp. olive oil
- ½ medium onion, diced
- 2 tsp. minced garlic
- 2 chicken breasts, chopped into pieces
  Vegetarians: 1 - 14 oz. can chickpeas, drained
- 2 tbsp. tomato paste
- 1 - 14 oz. can light coconut milk
- 2 tbsp. curry powder
- 1 tsp. chili powder
- 1 tbsp. ginger powder
- Salt and pepper, to taste

In a pan, heat the oil and sauté the onions and garlic until they are translucent. Add chicken, season with salt and pepper, and cook until the chicken turns white, about 7 minutes. (For vegetarians, add chickpeas instead of chicken and then move on to the next step.) Stir in coconut milk, spices, and tomato paste. Bring to a boil. Reduce heat to a simmer, and cook for another 7 - 10 minutes, stirring occasionally. Add salt and pepper to taste. Allow to sit for a few minutes before serving with your rice.

TURKEY MEATLOAF

Ingredients

- 1 lb. ground turkey
- 1 medium red onion, fine diced
- 4 ribs celery, fine diced
- 1 tbsp. olive oil
- 2 medium apples, tart
- 3 slices whole grain bread, crumbed
- ¾ cup Parmesan cheese, shredded
- 2½ tsp. poultry seasoning
- 2 whole eggs
- ¼ cup skim milk

In a large bowl, mix together the breadcrumbs, cheese, poultry seasoning, eggs, milk, cooled apple mixture, and turkey. Mix for no more than 2 minutes to keep it from getting tough. Place into a 9-inch greased loaf pan and bake in the oven for 45 minutes, or until the center is cooked through.

BBQ CHICKEN SALAD

Ingredients

- 3 chicken breasts, grilled or bbq, diced
- 6 cups romaine, chopped
- 1 tomato, diced
- ¾ cup canned corn (optional)
- ¾ cup canned black beans, drained & rinsed
- ¼ cup sweet or red onion, diced
- ¼ cup Monterey Jack cheese, shredded
- ½ cup Cheddar cheese, shredded
- ¼ cup Lite Ranch dressing
- ¼ cup BBQ sauce
- Tortilla chips, crushed

Place romaine into a bowl, top with diced chicken. Add vegetables and cheese. Combine Ranch dressing and BBQ sauce, pour over salad. Top with crushed tortilla chips.

MEXICAN STUFFED CHICKEN

SERVES: 4

Ingredients

- 4 chicken breasts, boneless/skinless
- 2 tbsp. dried whole grain breadcrumbs
- 2 tbsp. Parmesan cheese, grated
- 2 oz. Monterey Jack cheese cut into two slices, 3 inches by 1 inch
- 4 tbsp. mild green chilies, chopped
- 1 tsp. chili powder
- 2 eggs, beaten

Preheat oven to 375 degrees. Cut the chicken breast to ¼ inch thick. On each one, place a tablespoon of the chilies and a slice of Monterey Jack cheese. Roll up and place, seam side down, in a baking dish. Brush with beaten egg. Mix together the bread crumbs, Parmesan cheese, and chili powder and sprinkle over the chicken rolls, patting into place to form a crust. Bake for about 20 minutes – cheese inside will be melted and the crust nicely browned.

CHICKEN STEW

SERVES: 4

Ingredients

- 2 chicken breasts, whole
- 2 cups water
- 1 celery stalk, cut into 2" pieces
- ¼ onion, medium
- ½ green pepper, diced
- ½ lb. zucchini, diced
- ½ clove garlic, crushed
- 1 14-oz. can tomatoes, with juice (low sodium)
- 1 tsp. curry powder
- ¼ tsp. dried thyme
- ½ tsp. salt
- Dash cayenne pepper
- 1 tsp. olive oil
- ½ bay leaf

Place chicken in a medium pan with water, bay leaf, celery and ½ tsp. salt. Bring to a boil, reduce heat and simmer 20 minutes or until chicken is tender. Refrigerate chicken in broth overnight, or until fat is fully solid. Remove every trace of fat. Cut chicken into bite-sized pieces, discarding the skin. Save 1 cup of broth. In the same pot, sauté onion, peppers, garlic, and seasonings in the oil for a few minutes. Add tomatoes, zucchini, and broth and simmer 5 minutes, until zucchini is tender. Add chicken and heat through.

QUICK CHICKEN GUMBO

Ingredients

- 1 rotisserie chicken (approx. 2½ pounds), skin and bones removed, meat shredded (approx. 4 cups)
- 8 oz. turkey sausage, smoked (precooked), halved lengthwise and sliced 1" thick
- 3 tbsp. olive oil
- ⅓ cup whole grain flour
- 1 package cut okra (10 ounces) frozen
- 2 red bell peppers (ribs and seeds removed), chopped
- 1 medium onion, chopped
- 4 garlic cloves, chopped
- 1 tsp. dried oregano
- Coarse salt and ground pepper
- 4 cups water

In a 5-quart pot, heat oil over medium. Add flour and cook, whisking constantly, until pale golden, 5 to 7 minutes. Stir in bell peppers, onion, garlic, and oregano; season with salt and pepper. Cook, stirring occasionally, until vegetables are crisp-tender, 10 to 12 minutes.

Add 4 cups water; stir in okra and sausage. Bring to a boil. Stir in shredded chicken, and warm through, 1 to 2 minutes. Season with salt and pepper. Serve with cornbread.

TURKEY KABOBS

SERVES: 6

Ingredients

- 1 5-6 lb. frozen turkey breast, thawed
- 1 bunch green onions, sliced
- ¼ cup soy sauce
- ¼ cup dry sherry
- ¼ cup peach or tangerine jam
- 1 tbsp. fresh ginger, minced
- 1 tsp. salad oil
- ½ tsp. crushed red pepper

Mix the soy sauce, sherry, ginger, oil, jam, and red pepper in a large bowl. Cut the turkey from the bone and cut into 2-inch cubes. Add to the marinade and toss to coat well. Cover and refrigerate for several hours or overnight. Thread the turkey cubes onto metal skewers, alternating with onion pieces, then grill on a barbecue or in the oven for about 30 minutes, turning occasionally and brushing with marinade.

MUSHROOM & WILD RICE BLACK BEAN BURGER

MAKES: **10 BURGERS**

Ingredients

- 1 small onion, diced
- 3 large carrots, peeled and diced
- 2 cloves garlic, minced
- 2 cups portabella mushrooms, chopped
- 1 cup cooked wild rice
- 4 cups black beans (about 2-14.5 ounce cans), divided
- 1½ cup whole grain breadcrumbs
- ¼ cup fresh parsley, minced
- 1 tbsp. mustard
- 1 tbsp. chili powder
- 1½ tsp. salt
- 3 tbsp. olive oil
- 2 eggs

Heat the olive oil over medium-high heat in a large skillet. Add the onion, carrots, and garlic and cook until tender and fragrant, about five minutes. Add the mushrooms and cook until they release almost all of their water, about 10 minutes. Remove from heat and set aside.

In a food processor, combine the wild rice and three cups of the black beans. Pulse until it resembles a chunky paste. (Or smash with a fork/ potato smasher). In a large bowl, mix together the mushroom mixture, the rice mixture, the remaining black beans, and all remaining ingredients until well combined. Cover and refrigerate for a half hour.

Preheat oven to 350°. Line a baking sheet with parchment paper, set aside.

Form the chilled mixture into 10 even patties. Place on the prepared baking sheet and bake in preheated oven for 20-25 minutes, flipping them halfway through, or until the outsides are just barely golden brown.

SALMON STEAK FLORENTINE

SERVES: 4

Ingredients

- 4 4-oz. salmon steaks
- 2 bunches of fresh spinach (or use package of frozen spinach)
- 1 medium onion, chopped
- 1 clove garlic, chopped (optional)
- 2 lemons, cut into wedges
- 1 tsp. dried dill or 2 tsp. fresh
- 4 tsp. olive oil
- ¼ tsp. salt
- Pinch of pepper

Wash the spinach carefully and shake off water. Cut into 1-inch strips. Wipe fish with a damp cloth and arrange in a single layer on a broiler pan. Broil about 4 inches from the heat for 5 minutes. Turn, sprinkle with salt and pepper and brush the tops lightly with 2 tsp. of oil. Sprinkle on the dill. Return to broiler for 5 minutes. Meanwhile, heat the remaining oil in a skillet. Cook onion and garlic until soft. Stir in the spinach, cover pan and cook over high heat for 3 minutes or until spinach is wilted and bright green, stirring occasionally. To serve, spoon spinach onto a warm platter and lay salmon steaks on top.

BBQ TUNA

SERVES: 4

Ingredients

- 1 lb. tuna, fresh or frozen (albacore is preferable)
- 4 oz. grapefruit juice concentrate
- 4 tsp. lime juice (or lemon)
- ½ tsp. salt
- ½ tsp. Tabasco sauce
- ½ tsp. dried thyme
- ½ tsp. mustard

Combine grapefruit concentrate, lime or lemon juice, salt, Tabasco, thyme, and mustard in a bowl. Marinate fish for 30 minutes. Cook over barbecue grill or in oven broiler for 15 minutes, turning several times and basting with marinade mixture. Fish is done when it flakes easily with a fork.

CHICKEN HARVEST SOUP

SERVES: 6-8

Ingredients

- ½ lb. chicken or turkey, cooked
- 1½ cups harvest soup mix
- 1 cup carrots, sliced or diced
- 1 cup celery, stalk and leaf, finely chopped
- 1 cup cabbage, shredded
- 1 cup tomatoes, diced
- 1 tsp. salt
- ¼ tsp. pepper
- 1 tsp. instant chicken broth or 1 bouillon cube
- 4 cups water

Place water and Harvest Soup Mix in a heavy pot and simmer 1 hour.

Add all other ingredients and simmer another hour.

Options: Make with smoked turkey sausage and add 1 cup of each, fresh diced apples and sweet potatoes, instead of tomatoes.

Other spices that can be added: savory, garlic, and tarragon.

STIR-FRIED FISH FILLETS

Ingredients

- ½ lb. firm white fish fillets
- 1 bunch broccoli, cut into florets
- 1 tsp. soy sauce
- 2 tsp. water
- ½ tsp. cornstarch
- 2 tsp. olive oil
- ½ tsp. sesame oil
- 1 slice fresh ginger, minced

Whisk water and cornstarch together, set aside. Heat 1 tsp. of oil in a skillet. Add the fish and ginger and cook, stirring very gently so that fish cooks evenly but doesn't come apart. When fish starts to turn white, remove from pan. Pre-cook the broccoli by placing it in a small amount of boiling water for a few minutes. Drain. Heat the remaining teaspoon of oil in the skillet and add the broccoli, stir-frying 1-2 minutes until just crisp. Return fish to pan, add the soy sauce and water/cornstarch mix, and heat through so that sauce thickens and coats the fish and broccoli.

Optional: At the last minute, sprinkle on the sesame oil.

SPICE-RUBBED CHICKEN OVER SAUTEED SPINACH AND WHOLE GRAINS

SERVES: 4

Ingredients

- 2 lbs. boneless/skinless chicken thighs or breast, diced
- 1 cup barley
- 1 (10 oz.) bag spinach leaves
- Parmesan cheese, grated
- Olive oil
- 2 tsp. paprika
- 1 tsp. chili powder
- 1 tsp. ground cumin
- 1 tsp. ground thyme
- ¾ tsp. salt
- 1 tsp. garlic powder
- ½ tsp. ground pepper
- 2 tbsp. Worcestershire sauce
- 1 tbsp. honey
- 2½ cups broth or water

Preheat grill to medium high heat. Lightly brush grill with oil.

* Start preparing grains now.

In a small bowl, stir together paprika, chili powder, cumin, thyme, salt, 1/2 tsp. garlic powder, and pepper.

Place the chicken thighs in a large bowl, sprinkle the spice mixture over the chicken and toss to coat.

Grill the chicken until it is just cooked through, 4 to 5 minutes per side.

In a small bowl, whisk together the Worcestershire and honey. Brush mixture over chicken while grilling.

Bring 1 cup barley and 21/2 cups water or broth to a boil. Reduce heat to a simmer; cook, covered, until tender and most of the liquid has been absorbed, 40 to 50 minutes. Let stand 5 minutes. Makes 33 1/2 cups.

Heat 1 tbsp. olive oil in a large skillet over medium heat. Add the spinach to the skillet and cover; allow to cook 5 minutes. Stir in 1/2 tsp. garlic powder and cover again for another 5 minutes; remove from heat. Sprinkle with Parmesan cheese to serve. Serve chicken over spinach and grains.

EASY VEGETARIAN CHILI

SERVES: 4

Ingredients

- 2 28-oz. cans of whole tomatoes and their juice (crush gently)
- 2 cans of white or kidney beans, drained and rinsed
- 2 cups corn, fresh or frozen
- 3 stalks celery, diced
- 2 peppers, diced
- 2 carrots, diced
- 1 large onion, diced
- 4 garlic cloves, finely minced
- 2 tbsp. cumin
- 1 tsp. oregano
- 1-3 tbsp. chili powder
- ¼-2 tsp. of chili flakes
- 2 tbsp. olive oil
- Salt to taste

Optional: ¼ cup prawn or chicken stock (to add richness of flavor)

Optional Toppings: sour cream, cheddar cheese, cilantro, diced avocados, or green onion.

Heat oil in a large pot over medium-high heat. Add onion and sauté for about 3 minutes. Add garlic and sauté 1 minute more. Add spices and cook, stirring for about 30 seconds.

Add peppers, carrots, and celery and cook for about 5 minutes, or until they just start to soften. Add tomatoes and juice and bring to a simmer. Once the chili begins to simmer, reduce the heat to medium-low. Keep to a low simmer with the lid off for 20 minutes, stirring occasionally.

Add beans and corn and return to a simmer. Cook for 5 more minutes or until the corn and beans have heated through. Salt to taste. Serve on its own or top with one (or all) of the toppings.

Misc.

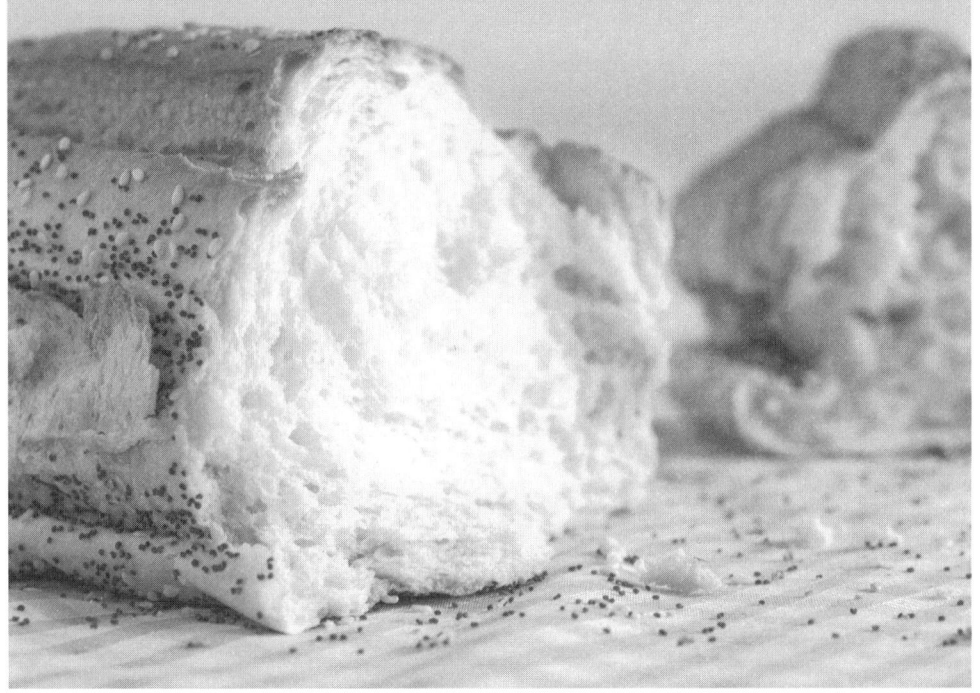

CHEWY GRANOLA BARS

Ingredients

- ½ cup raw or brown sugar
- 1½ cup honey
- ⅓ cup coconut oil
- ¼ tsp. salt
- 1 cup all natural peanut butter
- 2 tsp. vanilla

Heat the first 4 ingredients. Boil for 1 minute. Turn off the heat and add the peanut butter and vanilla. Set aside.

In a large bowl, combine:

- 4 cups crisp rice cereal
- 2 ⅔ cup quick oats
  (if you roll your own oats, toast them for 10 minutes at 350 degrees. Cool and then pulse in a food processor)
- 1/3 cup ground flax seed

Pour the hot mixture over the dry and stir to coat. Line a 12x15 pan with parchment paper. Pour in the granola and spread out. Top with another layer of parchment paper and press down with another 12x15 pan to compress the bars. Remove the top pan and paper. Sprinkle with ½-1 cup mini chocolate chips, raisins, or dried cranberries. Replace the paper and pan and press again. Allow the bars to cool completely, then cut and wrap. Store in the refrigerator.

CONDENSED TOMATO SOUP SUBSTITUTE

Ingredients

- 8 oz. tomato sauce
- 1-2 tbsp. sugar
- 1 tbsp. cornstarch
- ½ tsp. salt
- 1-2 tsp. ketchup

Whisk all together. One batch equals one can of condensed tomato soup.

NO-BAKE ENERGY BITES

Ingredients

- 1 cup quick oats
  (if you roll your own oats, toast them for 10 minutes at 350 degrees. Cool and then pulse in a food processor)
- ½ cup chopped coconut
- ½ cup all natural creamy peanut butter
- ¼ cup ground flax seed
- ½ cup honey
- 1 tsp. vanilla
- ¼ cup oat bran
- 2 tbsp. flax seed or 1 tbsp. chia seeds
- ½ cup mini chocolate chips

Mix all together. Refrigerate 1 hour. Roll into walnut sized balls and store in an airtight container in the refrigerator.

For kids, 1-2 of these a day helps with regularity

WHOLE-GRAIN BREAD

Ingredients

- 1½ cups hot water
- ⅓ cup olive oil
- ⅓ cup honey
- 2 tsp. salt
- 1 egg
- 2 tbsp. liquid lecithin
- 4-4 ½ cups freshly milled flour (Prairie Gold is delicious)
- 1 tbsp. instant yeast
- ¼ cup ground flaxseed (optional)

Combine the water, oil, honey, salt, and egg in a mixer. Add the lecithin and flaxseed. Add the flour one cup at a time, stirring well after each one to make a soft dough. Knead 5-6 minutes. Add a little more flour if needed, you want the dough to pull away from the sides. Let rise, covered, until double (about one hour in a warm place). Shape into 2 loaves and place into two loaf pans brushed with a 50/50 mix of olive oil and liquid lecithin. Let rise (uncovered) until the tops of the loaves are just above the rim of the pan (about one hour in a warm place). Bake at 350 degrees for 25-30 minutes or until the tops and bottoms are golden. Remove from pans immediately and cool on a wire rack.

BASIC CREAM SOUP

Replaces cream of mushroom or other soups in casseroles.

Ingredients

- 3 tbsp. butter
- 3 tbsp. finely ground white bean flour
  (can use whole grain or all-purpose flour, the bean flour is an additional source of protein)
- 1½ tsp. chicken bouillon
- ½ tsp. salt
- ¼ tsp. pepper
- 1½ cups milk

In a saucepan over medium heat, melt the butter and brown slightly. Add the bouillon, salt, and pepper. Stir. Add the flour and stir constantly for about a minute to cook the flour. Slowly add the milk, stirring constantly until smooth. Allow to heat, stirring constantly until thickened. One batch of this soup equals a can of cream soup.

* For mushroom soup, add ¼ cup chopped fresh mushrooms along with the butter.

* For celery soup, add ¼ cup finely diced cooked celery.

* For more flavorful soup, add 2 tbsp. finely diced onion along with the butter.

HOMEMADE SOFT TORTILLAS

Ingredients

- 1 cup whole grain flour (grinding your own Prairie Gold wheat berries is best)
- 1 cup all-purpose flour
- 1 cup warm milk
- 1 tsp. salt
- 1 tbsp. olive oil
- 1½ tsp. baking powder

Combine all and mix well. Turn onto a floured surface and knead. Divide into 10 balls and place onto a cookie sheet. Cover with a moist towel and allow to rest 30 minutes. To cook each one, roll out very thin and then cook for 1-2 minutes per side on a hot griddle or pan sprayed lightly with olive oil or cooking spray.

Recipe Index

3 Ingredient Pancakes 81
Almond Butter Banana Oatmeal Smoothie 79
Apple-Berry Smoothie 80
Bakked French Fries 91
Basic Cream Soup 113
BBQ Chicken Salad 102
BBQ Tuna 106
Blackened Fish Tacos w/ Avocado-Cilantro Sauce 85
Breakfast Casserole 82
Broiled Shrimp with Lemon 100
Brown Sugar BBQ Salmon 90
Chewy Granola Bars 111
Chicken Burgers 89
Chicken Burritos 92
Chicken Harvest Soup 107
Chicken Stew 103
Chicken Stir-Fry 89
Chicken, Brussels Sprouts and Quinoa Salad 84
Chopped Avocado, Feta and Barley Salad 87
Condensed Tomato Soup Substitute 111
Cucumber Salmon Salad 87
Curried Tuna Salad Sandwich 84
Easy Vegetarian Chili 109
Eggplant Lasagna 94
Eggplant Parmesan 93
Healthy Fried Rice 96
Healthy Yummasetti 93
Homemade Soft Tortillas 113

Lemon-Basil Butter Chicken 97
Mashed Cauliflower 92
Mexican Stuffed Chicken 102
Mushroom & Wild Rice Black Bean Burger 105
No-Bake Energy Bites 112
Quick and Easy Granola 80
Quick Chicken Gumbo 104
Salmon Steak Florentine 106
Sesame-Roasted Turnips and Barley 98
Side Salad with Quinoa 87
Simple Chicken Curry 101
Soy Salmon with Stir-Fried Quinoa 99
Spice-Rubbed Chicken Over Sauteed Spinach & Whole Grains 108
Spinach and Feta Pie with Chickpea Flour Crust 100
Stir-Fried Fish Filet 107
Strawberry Avocado Spinach Salad with Chicken 86
Sweet Potato Fries 95
Tomato and White Bean Soup 97
Tomato Spinach Pasta 90
Turkey Kabobs 104
Turkey Meatloaf 101
Vegetable Bean Fajitas 96
Vegetable Pizza 95
Veggie Couscous 91
Whole-Grain Bread 112
Whole-Grain Pancakes 79

PART TWO
EXERCISE

For the Love of Living

Chapter Five
INTRODUCTION TO EXERCISE

What is the reason that you turned to this page? Is it because you want to learn more about exercise, already love exercise and want to improve, want to lose weight, or have always felt that exercise was just not for you? Whatever the reason, this handbook is for you.

Exercise is for everyone, including children and older adults. It is for individuals with physical impairments, or for those who struggle with weight problems (and even those who don't). (It is recommended to consult your physician for specific recommendations for your condition). The benefits of exercise are endless! They range from better mood and energy to increased brainpower and a longer life.

The good news is that incorporating exercise into our daily lifestyle can be easy and fun. Experts recommend doing physical activity that you enjoy, starting out slowly.

We have included detailed information on the many benefits of physical activity for both the young and the not-so-young, as well as recommendations for how to supplement nutrition with exercise. If getting started sounds intimidating to you, we've got a lot of solutions and advice on where to begin, based on your current activity level. You will find instructions for beginners and for those who are more experienced in exercise. These instructions include stretching, strength training, running, everyday exercises, and family fitness. If you're looking to exercise to help you lose weight, look for some helpful and proven tips in the Exercising to Lose Weight section.

We hope that this handbook will inspire and equip you to add exercise to your life. Here's to a better you!

For the Love of Living

Chapter Six

LEARNING ABOUT EXERCISE

THE BENEFITS & IMPORTANCE OF EXERCISE[3]

Regular physical activity is one of the most important things you can do for your health. It can help:

- Control your weight
- Reduce your risk of cardiovascular disease
- Reduce your risk of type 2 diabetes and metabolic syndrome
- Reduce your risk of some cancers
- Strengthen your bones and muscles
- Improve your mental health and mood
- Improve your ability to do daily activities and prevent falls if you're an older adult
- Increase your chances of living longer

If you're not sure about becoming active or boosting your level of physical activity because you're afraid of getting hurt, the good news is that moderate-intensity aerobic activity, like brisk walking, is safe for most people.

Start slowly - Cardiac events such as a heart attack are rare during physical activity. But the risk does go up if you suddenly become much more active than usual. For example, you can put yourself at risk if you normally do not get much physical activity and then suddenly do vigorous-intensity aerobic activity, like shoveling snow. That's why it's important to start slowly, and gradually increase your level of activity.

If you have a chronic health condition such as arthritis, diabetes, or heart disease, talk with your doctor to find out if your condition limits your ability to be active. Work with your doctor to come up with a physical activity plan that matches your abilities. If your condition prevents you from meeting the minimum guidelines, try to do as much as you can. What's important is that you avoid being inactive. Even 60 minutes a week of moderate-intensity aerobic activity is good for you.

The bottom line is - the health benefits of physical activity far outweigh the risks of getting hurt.

CONTROL YOUR WEIGHT

Are you looking to get to or stay at a healthy weight? Both diet and physical activity play a critical role in controlling your weight. You gain weight when the calories you burn, including those burned during physical activity, are less than the calories you eat or drink. When it comes to weight management, people vary greatly in how much physical activity they need. You may need to be more active than others to achieve or maintain a healthy weight.

To maintain your weight: Work your way up to 150 minutes of

moderate-intensity aerobic activity, 75 minutes of vigorous-intensity aerobic activity, or an equivalent mix of the two each week. Scientific evidence shows that physical activity can help you maintain your weight over time. However, the exact amount of physical activity needed to do this is not clear since it varies widely from person to person. It's possible that you may need to do more than the equivalent of 150 minutes of moderate-intensity activity a week to maintain your weight.

To lose weight and keep it off: You will need a high amount of physical activity unless you also adjust your diet and reduce the number of calories you're taking in. Getting to and staying at a healthy weight requires both regular physical activity and a healthy eating plan. For more information see our section on Exercising to Lose Weight.

REDUCE YOUR RISK OF CARDIOVASCULAR DISEASE

Heart disease and stroke are two of the leading causes of death in the United States. Following the recommended guidelines and getting at least 150 minutes a week of moderate-intensity aerobic activity can put you at a lower risk for these diseases. You can reduce your risk even further with more physical activity. Regular physical activity can also lower your blood pressure and improve your cholesterol levels.

REDUCE YOUR RISK OF TYPE 2 DIABETES AND METABOLIC SYNDROME

Regular physical activity can reduce your risk of developing type 2 diabetes and metabolic syndrome. Metabolic syndrome is a condition in which you have some combination of too much fat around the waist, high blood pressure, low HDL cholesterol, high triglycerides, or high blood sugar. Research shows that lower rates of these conditions are seen with 120 to 150 minutes a week of at least moderate-intensity aerobic activity. The more physical activity you do, the lower your risk will be.

Already have type 2 diabetes? Regular physical activity can help control your blood glucose levels.

REDUCE YOUR RISK OF SOME CANCERS
Being physically active lowers your risk for two types of cancer: colon and breast cancer.

Research shows that:

- Physically active people have a lower risk of colon cancer than do people who are not active.

- Physically active women have a lower risk of breast cancer than women who are not active.

- Reduce your risk of endometrial and lung cancer. Although the research is not yet final, some findings suggest that your risk of endometrial cancer and lung cancer may be lower if you get regular physical activity compared to people who are not active.

Improve your quality of life. If you are a cancer survivor, research shows that getting regular physical activity not only helps give you a better quality of life, but also improves your physical fitness.

STRENGTHEN YOUR BONES AND MUSCLES
As you age, it's important to protect your bones, joints, and muscles. Not only do they support your body and help you move, but keeping them healthy can enhance your ability to do your daily activities and be physically active. Research shows that doing aerobic, muscle-strengthening and bone-strengthening physical activity of at least a moderately-intense level can slow the loss of bone density that comes with age.

Hip fracture is a serious health condition that can have life-changing negative effects, especially if you're an older adult. Research shows that people who do 120 to 300 minutes of at least moderate-intensity aerobic activity each week have a lower risk of hip fracture.

Regular physical activity helps with arthritis and other conditions affecting the joints. If you have arthritis, research shows that doing 130 to 150 minutes a week of moderate-intensity, low-impact aerobic activity can not only improve your ability to manage pain and do everyday tasks, but it can also make your quality of life better.

Build strong, healthy muscles. Muscle-strengthening activities can help you increase or maintain your muscle mass and strength. Slowly increasing the amount of weight and the number of repetitions that you do will give you even more benefits, no matter your age.

IMPROVE YOUR MENTAL HEALTH AND MOOD
Regular physical activity can help keep your thinking, learning, and judgment skills sharp. It can also reduce your risk of depression and may help you sleep better. Regular physical activity boosts your memory and the ability to learn new things as well. When you exercise, it increases production of cells in the hippocampus, a part of the brain responsible for memory and learning.[12] Research has shown that doing aerobic or a mix of aerobic and muscle-strengthening activities 3 to 5 times a week for 30 to 60 minutes can give you these mental health benefits. Some scientific evidence has also shown that even lower levels of physical activity can be beneficial.

IMPROVE YOUR ABILITY TO DO DAILY ACTIVITIES AND PREVENT FALLS
A functional limitation for those who are aging is a loss of the ability to do everyday activities such as climbing stairs, grocery shopping, or playing with your grandchildren.

How does this relate to physical activity? If you're a physically active middle-aged or older adult, you have a lower risk of functional limitations than people who are inactive

Already have trouble doing some of your everyday activities? Aerobic and muscle-strengthening activities can help improve your ability to do these types of tasks.

Are you an older adult who is at risk for falls? Research shows that doing balance and muscle-strengthening activities each week along with moderate-intensity aerobic activity, like brisk walking, can help reduce your risk of falling.

INCREASE YOUR CHANCES OF LIVING LONGER
Science shows that physical activity can reduce your risk of dying early from the leading causes of death, like heart disease and some cancers. This is remarkable in two ways:

1. Only a few lifestyle choices have as large an impact on your health as physical activity. People who are physically active for about 7 hours a week have a 40 percent lower risk of dying early than those who are active for less than 30 minutes a week.

2. You don't have to do high amounts of activity or vigorous-intensity activity to reduce your risk of premature death. You can put yourself at lower risk of dying early by doing at least 150 minutes a week of moderate-intensity aerobic activity.

Everyone can gain the health benefits of physical activity - age, ethnicity, shape, or size do not matter.

In addition to the health benefits listed above, moderate exercise, like brisk walking, can have other health benefits such as:
- Improves blood circulation (which reduces the risk of heart disease)
- Improves your sleep - help you fall asleep faster and sleep more soundly
- Improves blood cholesterol levels
- Prevents and manages high blood pressure
- Prevents bone loss
- Boosts energy levels

- Increases productivity
- Helps manage stress
- Releases tension/ reduces stress
- Promotes enthusiasm and optimism
- Counters anxiety and depression
- Helps control addiction
- Improves self-image
- Reduces risk of stroke by 20 percent in moderately active people and by 27 percent in those who are highly active
- Establishes good heart-healthy habits in children and counters the conditions (obesity, high blood pressure, poor cholesterol levels, poor lifestyle habits, etc.) that lead to heart attack and stroke later in life

And that's not all. Being more active can:
- Be fun
- Be a way to enjoy the outdoors
- Help you look your best
- Help you feel better about yourself
- Increase creative thinking
- Provides a way to share an activity with family and friends
- Inspire others

HEALTH BENEFITS FOR SENIORS[4]

Being inactive can be risky. Although exercise and physical activity are among the healthiest things you can do for yourself, some older adults are reluctant to get started. Some are afraid that exercise will be too hard or that physical activity will harm them. Others might think they have to join a gym or have special equipment. However, studies show that "taking it easy" is risky. For the most part, when older people lose their ability to do things on their own, it doesn't happen just because they've aged; it's frequently because they're not active. Lack of physical activity also can lead to more visits to the doctor, more hospitalizations, and more use of medicines for a variety of illnesses.

Scientists have found that staying physically active and exercising on a regular basis can help prevent or delay many diseases and disabilities. In some cases, exercise is an effective treatment for chronic conditions. For example, studies show that people with arthritis, heart disease, or diabetes benefit from regular exercise. It also helps people with high blood pressure, balance problems, or difficulty walking.

HOW MUCH EXERCISE DO I NEED FOR MY AGE & CONDITION?

According to the Centers for Disease Control and Prevention, the following levels of activities are recommended for each age group in America.

ADULTS NEED AT LEAST:

Walking - 150 minutes of moderate-intensity aerobic activity (i.e., brisk walking) every week and -

Weight training/muscle-strengthening activities on 2 or more days a week that work all major muscle groups (legs, hips, back, abdomen, chest, shoulders, and arms).

OR

Jogging - 75 minutes of vigorous-intensity aerobic activity (i.e., jogging or running) every week and -

Weight training/muscle-strengthening activities on 2 or more days a week that work all major muscle groups (legs, hips, back, abdomen, chest, shoulders, and arms).

OR

An equivalent mix of moderate and vigorous-intensity aerobic activity and -

Weight training/muscle-strengthening activities on 2 or more days a week that work all major muscle groups (legs, hips, back, abdomen, chest, shoulders, and arms).

CHILDREN

Children and adolescents should do 60 minutes or more of physical activity each day.

This may sound like a lot, but don't worry, your child may already be meeting the physical activity guidelines. You will soon discover all the easy and enjoyable ways to help your child meet the recommendations.

Encourage your child to participate in activities that are age-appropriate, enjoyable, and offer variety. Just make sure your child or adolescent is doing three types of physical activity:

1. Aerobic Activity

   Aerobic activity should make up most of your child's 60 or more minutes of physical activity each day. This can include either moderate-intensity aerobic activity such as brisk walking, or vigorous-intensity activity such as running. Be sure to include vigorous-intensity aerobic activity on at least 3 days per week.

2. Muscle Strengthening

   Include muscle-strengthening activities such as gymnastics or push-ups at least 3 days per week as part of your child's 60 or more minutes.

3. Bone-Strengthening

   Include bone-strengthening activities such as jumping rope or running at least 3 days per week as part of your child's 60 or more minutes.

What do you mean by "age-appropriate" activities?
Some physical activity is better suited for children than adolescents. For example, children do not normally need formal muscle-strengthening programs, such as lifting weights. Younger children usually strengthen their muscles when they do gymnastics, play on a jungle gym, or climb trees. As children grow older and become adolescents, they may start structured weight programs. For example, they may do these types of programs along with their football or basketball team practice.

OLDER ADULTS
As an older adult, regular physical activity is one of the most important things you can do for your health. It can prevent many of the health problems that seem to come with age. It also helps your muscles grow stronger so that you can keep doing your day-to-day activities without becoming dependent on others.

Not doing any physical activity can be bad for you, no matter your age or health condition. Keep in mind; some physical activity is better than none at all. You will also increase the benefits to your health as you step up your physical activity. If you're 65 years of age or older, are generally fit and have no limiting health conditions, you can follow the guidelines listed below.

For important health benefits, older adults need at least the same amount of activity as that recommended for younger adults, 10 minutes at a time is fine.

We know that 150 minutes each week sounds like a lot of time, but it's not. That's 2 hours and 30 minutes; about the same amount of time you might spend watching a movie. The good news is that you can spread out your activity during the week, so you don't have to do it all at once. You can even break it up into smaller chunks of time during the day. It's about what works best for you, as long as you're doing physical activity at moderate or vigorous effort for at least 10 minutes at a time.

For even greater health benefits, older adults should increase their activity to:

Jogging - 300 minutes each week of moderate-intensity aerobic activity and -

Weight training/muscle-strengthening activities on 2 or more days a week that work all major muscle groups (legs, hips, back, abdomen, chest, shoulders, and arms).

OR

Jogging - 150 minutes each week of vigorous-intensity aerobic activity and -

Weight training/muscle-strengthening activities on 2 or more days a week that work all major muscle groups (legs, hips, back, abdomen, chest, shoulders, and arms).

OR

Walking/jogging - An equivalent mix of moderate and vigorous-intensity aerobic activity and -

Weight training/muscle-strengthening activities on 2 or more days a week that work all major muscle groups (legs, hips, back, abdomen, chest, shoulders, and arms).

PREGNANT/POSTPARTUM WOMEN

Is it okay to be physically active while I'm pregnant and after I have my baby?

Yes! If you are a healthy pregnant or postpartum woman, physical activity is good for your overall health. For example, moderate-intensity physical activity such as brisk walking keeps your heart and lungs healthy during and after pregnancy. Physical activity also helps improve your mood throughout the postpartum period. After you have your baby, exercise helps maintain a healthy weight and when combined with eating fewer calories, helps with weight loss.

According to the 2008 Physical Activity Guidelines for Americans, healthy women should get at least 150 minutes per week of moderate-intensity aerobic activity, such as brisk walking, during and after their pregnancy. It is best to spread this activity throughout the week.

Healthy women who already do a vigorous-intensity aerobic activity such as running, or large amounts of activity, can continue doing so during and after their pregnancy, provided they stay healthy. They should discuss with their health-care provider about how and when to adjust the activity over time, 10 minutes at a time is fine.

Aren't there risks involved with physical activity and pregnancy?
According to scientific evidence, the risks of moderate-intensity aerobic activity such as brisk walking are very low for healthy pregnant women. Physical activity does not increase your chances of low birth weight, early delivery, or early pregnancy loss. It's also not likely that the composition or amount of your breast milk or your baby's growth will be affected by physical activity.

What are some things to keep in mind when I do physical activity during and after my pregnancy?
Unless you have a medical reason to avoid physical activity during or after your pregnancy, you can begin or continue moderate-intensity aerobic activity. You can find more information on moderate-intensity activity in the Active Adults section. If you begin physical activity during your pregnancy, start slowly and increase your amount gradually over time. While pregnant, you should avoid doing any activity that involves lying on your back or that puts you at risk of falling or incurring abdominal injury, such as horseback riding, soccer, or basketball.

If meeting the recommendations for exercise sounds out of reach for you, you're in luck. Continue reading for suggestions on the hesitations and barriers that keep many people from exercising, including time, willpower, and resources.

Don't give up yet! Exercise is for everyone and can be fun. You can do it!

ACTIVITIES & LEVELS OF EXERTION[3]

The American Heart Association's recommendation for adult physical activity is a combination of at least 150 minutes of moderate exercise or 75 minutes of vigorous exercise per week.

So how exactly do we measure moderate and vigorous exercise to know if we're working out at the right intensity?

There are a couple of different ways to measure the level of intensity at which you are exercising, and that level is based on your individual fitness level and overall health.

PERCEIVED EXERTION *(Borg Rating of Perceived Exertion Scale)*
The Borg Rating of Perceived Exertion (RPE) is a way of measuring physical activity intensity level. Perceived exertion is how hard you feel like your body is working. It is based on the physical sensations a person experiences during physical activity, including increased heart rate, increased respiration or breathing rate, increased sweating, and muscle fatigue. Although this is a subjective measure, a person's exertion rating may provide a fairly good estimate of the actual heart rate during physical activity* (Borg, 1998).

Practitioners generally agree that perceived exertion ratings between 12 to 14 on the Borg Scale suggests that physical activity is being performed at a moderate level of intensity. During an activity, use the Borg Scale to assign numbers to how you feel (see instructions below). Self-monitoring how hard your body is working can help you adjust the intensity of the activity by speeding up or slowing down your movements.

Through the experience of monitoring how your body feels, it will become easier to know when to adjust your intensity. For example, a walker who wants to engage in moderate-intensity activity would aim for a Borg Scale level of "somewhat hard" (12-14). If he describes his muscle fatigue and breathing as "very light" (9 on the Borg Scale) he would want to increase his intensity. On the other hand, if he felt his exertion was "extremely hard" (19 on the Borg Scale) he would need to slow down his movements to achieve the moderate-intensity range.

*A high correlation exists between a person's perceived exertion rating times 10 and the actual heart rate during physical activity; so a person's exertion rating may provide a fairly good estimate of the actual heart rate during activity (Borg, 1998). For example, if a person's rating of perceived exertion (RPE) is 12, then 12 x 10 = 120; so the heart rate should be approximately 120 beats per minute. Note that this calculation is only an approximation of heart rate, and the actual heart rate can vary quite a bit depending on age and physical condition. The Borg Rating of Perceived Exertion is also the preferred method to assess intensity among those individuals who take medications that affect heart rate or pulse.

INSTRUCTIONS FOR BORG RATING OF PERCEIVED EXERTION (RPE) SCALE

While doing physical activity, we want you to rate your perception of exertion. This feeling should reflect how heavy and strenuous the exercise feels to you, combining all sensations and feelings of physical stress, effort, and fatigue. Do not concern yourself with any one factor such as leg pain or shortness of breath, but try to focus on your total feeling of exertion.

Look at the rating scale below while you are engaging in an activity; it ranges from 6 to 20, where 6 means "no exertion at all" and 20 means "maximal exertion." Choose the number from below that best describes your level of exertion. This will give you a good idea of the intensity level of your activity, and you can use this information to speed up or slow down your movements to reach your desired range.

Try to appraise your feeling of exertion as honestly as possible, without thinking about what the actual physical load is. Your own feeling of effort and exertion is important, not how it compares to other people's. Look at the scales and the expressions and then give a number.

EXAMPLES

9 corresponds to "very light" exercise. For a healthy person, it is like walking slowly at his or her own pace for some minutes. You would most likely be able to sing during this level of activity.

6	NO EXERTION AT ALL
7	
7.5	EXTREMELY LIGHT
8	
9	VERY LIGHT
10	
11	LIGHT
12	
13	SOMEWHAT HARD
14	
15	HARD (HEAVY)
16	
17	VERY HARD
18	
19	EXTREMELY HARD
20	MAXIMAL EXERTION

13 on the scale is "somewhat hard" exercise, but it still feels OK to continue. You would most likely be able to talk, but not sing during this level of activity.

17 "very hard" is very strenuous. A healthy person can still go on, but he or she really has to push him - or herself. It feels very heavy, and the person is very tired. You would most likely not be able to say more than a few words without pausing for a breath during this level.

19 on the scale is an extremely strenuous exercise level. For most people, this is the most strenuous exercise they have ever experienced.

LOW-INTENSITY EXERCISE
The Centers for Disease Control and Prevention puts physical activity on a spectrum based on heart rate and physical exertion. Light exercise is the lowest end of the spectrum but is still good for your health. Low-level activity, relative to ones individual capacity, would rate 9-11 on the Borg scale.

Examples of low-intensity exercise:
- Walking slowly
- Cooking
- Vacuuming
- Light Gardening
- Dusting
- Golfing, using a cart to travel between holes

You can easily turn light exercise into moderate-intensity activity by increasing the speed or duration.

MODERATE-INTENSITY EXERCISE
Moderate level activity, relative to ones individual capacity, would rate 12-14 on the Borg scale.

Learning About Exercise

Recommendations for Moderate Level Activity

Your exercise can be done all at one time, or intermittently throughout the day. Activities to get you started could include walking or swimming at a slow pace. You can start out by walking 30 minutes for 3 days a week and build to 45 minutes of more intense walking at least 5 days a week. With this plan, you can burn 100 to 200 more calories per day. All adults should set a long-term goal to accumulate at least 30 minutes or more of moderate-intensity physical activity on most, and preferably all, days of the week. This regimen can be adapted to other forms of physical activity, but walking is particularly attractive because of its safety and accessibility. Also, try to increase "everyday" activity like taking the stairs instead of the elevator. Reducing sedentary time is a good strategy to increase activity by undertaking frequent, less strenuous activities. With time, you may be able to engage in more strenuous activities. Competitive sports such as tennis and volleyball can provide an enjoyable form of exercise for many, but care must be taken to avoid injury.

Examples of moderate-intensity exercise:

Common Chores
- Washing and waxing a car for 45–60 minutes
- Washing windows or floors for 45–60 minutes
- Gardening for 30–45 minutes
- Wheeling self in wheelchair for 30–40 minutes
- Pushing a stroller 1.5 miles in 30 minutes
- Raking leaves for 30 minutes
- Walking 2 miles in 30 minutes (15 min/mile)
- Shoveling snow for 15 minutes
- Stair walking for 15 minutes

Sporting Activities
- Playing volleyball for 45–60 minutes
- Playing touch football for 45 minutes

- Walking 1.75 miles in 35 minutes (20 min/mile)
- Basketball (shooting baskets) for 30 minutes
- Bicycling 5 miles in 30 minutes
- Water aerobics for 30 minutes
- Swimming laps for 20 minutes
- Basketball (playing game) for 15–20 minutes
- Bicycling 4 miles in 15 minutes
- Jumping rope for 15 minutes
- Running 1.5 miles in 15 minutes (10 min/mile)

VIGOROUS-INTENSITY EXERCISE

Vigorous activity is a level that requires the highest amount of oxygen consumption to complete the activity. Relative to an individual's personal capacity, vigorous-intensity physical activity is usually 17-19 on the Borg scale.

Examples of vigorous-intensity exercise:
- Race walking, jogging, or running
- Swimming laps
- Tennis (singles)
- Heavy gardening (digging, hoeing)
- Bicycling 10 miles per hour or faster
- Jumping rope
- Heavy gardening (continuous digging or hoeing)
- Hiking uphill or with a heavy backpack
- Sports with a lot of running (basketball, hockey, soccer)

AEROBIC ACTIVITY – WHAT COUNTS?

Aerobic activity or "cardio" gets you breathing harder and your heart beating faster. From pushing a lawn mower to biking to the store – all types of activities count as long as you're doing them at a moderate or vigorous intensity for at least 10 minutes at a time. Even something as simple as walking is a great way to get the aerobic activity you need, as long as it's at a moderately intense pace.

EXERCISE & NUTRITION

Do you wonder what you should eat to fuel up for exercise, or how nutrition and exercise work together for your overall health and weight loss?

Exercise and nutrition go hand in hand when it comes to our health and should be a fundamental part of everyone's lives. It is important to note that exercising while ignoring your diet is not wholly beneficial, and neither is giving high attention to your diet and ignoring exercise.

Some think that if they exercise regularly, they can eat whatever they want and not gain weight. Is this true? No; although some active people may be able to keep weight off and still eat high-calorie diets, their ability to do so is more likely due to a rapid metabolism rather than exercise alone. Many people overestimate the number of calories burned while working out, which is usually significantly less than a food splurge. Exercise should be accompanied with recommended portion sizes and healthy eating guidelines. Those who are engaging in a serious activity such as a triathlon should increase their calorie intake. However, for the casual exerciser working out for an hour or less at a time, a healthy balanced diet and portion recommendations will usually suffice.

Knowing when and what to eat can make an impact in the way you feel and perform during exercise. Consider the following tips.

WHAT TO EAT
Your body needs extra energy if you are planning to exercise. The best types of food for this energy are usually complex carbohydrates (whole grains) and proteins. Carbohydrates fuel workouts. Protein helps repair and build muscle after exercising.

WHEN TO EAT

The general guideline:
- Large meals. Eat these at least three to four hours before exercising.
- Small meals. Eat these two to three hours before exercising.
- Small snacks. Eat these an hour before exercising.

Eating too much before you exercise can leave you feeling sluggish. Eating too little might not give you the energy to keep you feeling strong throughout your workout.

EXERCISING IN THE MORNING
- What you ate the previous day will have used most of its energy by morning and your blood sugar level may be low. This might make you feel sluggish or lightheaded when you exercise.

- Include time to get up and eat at least 1.5 hours before exercising. This will give you enough time to digest the food and use its energy.

- If you prefer a light breakfast before exercise, you can eat an hour beforehand and choose something that will raise your blood sugar such as fruit or juice and a simple carbohydrate.

GOOD BREAKFAST OPTIONS INCLUDE:
- Whole-grain cereals or bread
- Peanut Butter (with toast or fruit)
- Low-fat milk
- Bananas
- Yogurt
- Eggs

If you normally have coffee in the morning, a cup before your workout is ok. Remember that anytime you try a food or drink for the first time before a workout, you risk an upset stomach. Also, be careful not to overeat before exercise.

EXERCISE IN-BETWEEN MEALS

If you're exercising several hours after your main meal or in between meals it is important to grab a healthy snack about an hour before you begin. Eating shortly before exercising may not give you extra energy but will help prevent a blood sugar swing during the activity.

Good snack options include:
- Energy bars
- Bananas or other fresh fruit
- Yogurt
- Fruit smoothies
- Whole-grain bagel or crackers
- Low-fat granola bars
- Peanut butter sandwiches
- Hard-boiled egg

POST-EXERCISE NUTRITION

Your body uses stored energy (glycogen) in your muscles to fuel your workout, so it is important, after finishing, to replenish the nutrients lost. You also need to rehydrate after working out, so drink plenty of water. To help your muscles recover and to replace their glycogen stores, eat a meal or snack that contains both protein and carbohydrates within two hours of your exercise session, if possible. If you are planning to eat a meal within a couple of hours after exercising, there is no need to have a post-exercise snack.

Good post-workout food choices include:
- Smoothie (with low-fat milk and fruit)
- Low-fat chocolate milk and pretzels
- Peanut butter sandwich
- Yogurt and fruit (especially berries)
- Cheese and whole-grain crackers
- Pasta with meatballs
- Chicken with brown rice

- Turkey on a whole-grain wrap with veggies

These options are quick and convenient and offer carbs and some protein. The liquid from the first two choices will help rehydrate the body.

HYDRATION

Hydration is one of the most important elements of a good workout. Did you know that your muscle tissue is comprised of 75% water? Therefore, it is important not to forget to drink water to fuel an exercise. You need adequate fluids before, during, and after exercise to help prevent dehydration.

An easy-to-remember rule for daily water intake is 8 – 8oz glasses of fluid a day.

To stay well-hydrated for exercise, the American College of Sports Medicine recommends that you:

- Drink roughly 2 to 3 cups (473 to 710 milliliters) of water during the two to three hours before your workout.

- Drink about 1/2 to 1 cup (118 to 237 milliliters) of water every 15 to 20 minutes during your workout. Adjust amounts related to your body size and the weather.

- Drink roughly 2 to 3 cups (473 to 710 milliliters) of water after your workout for every pound of weight you lose during the workout.

The most important thing is to learn to recognize when you are dehydrated. Every person is different and should eat and drink according to what their body needs.

"The secret of getting ahead is getting started."
-Mark Twain

"If you always put limits on everything you do, physical or anything else, it will spread into your work and into your life. There are no limits. There are only plateaus; and you must not stay there, you must go beyond them."
- Bruce Lee

"I've missed more than 9,000 shots in my career. I've lost almost 300 games. 26 times, I've been trusted to take the game winning shot and missed. I've failed over and over and over again in my life. And that is why I succeed."
-Michael Jordan

"Start simply, but simply start."
–Tammy Maltby

Chapter Seven
GETTING STARTED

Are you ready to get started exercising? Is there something holding you back? Use the following questionnaires from the Centers for Disease Control and Prevention (CDC) to help you assess where you're at and then get started. Remember that exercise is for everyone. Choose activities that you enjoy and start slowly, and you are bound to have fun and reap the benefits!

How active are you now?[2]
1. There are things holding me back.
2. I'm just getting started.
3. I'm doing a little, but I'm ready to get more active.
4. I'm already physically active, and I want to keep it up.

The following tips are meant for adults. See the Everyday Exercise for the Whole Family section for ways to encourage kids to get active.

THERE ARE THINGS HOLDING ME BACK

Hurdle: It's been a long time since I've been physically active.

Solution: Choose something small, such as walking, to get started. Be sure to pick something that you enjoy. Do a little at a time and add as you go. Before long you will be at a very active level again.

Hurdle: I don't have time.

Solution: Start small. The CDC suggests that you can do 10 minutes at a time if you are pressed for time or energy. Take a walk or get active during your lunch break, do some jumping jacks, or walk up and down a staircase while waiting on something at home. These 10-minute intervals add up.

Hurdle: It costs too much.

Solution: You don't need expensive equipment or a club membership to exercise. There are many ways to do exercises at home using household items, as well as introducing more activity into your lifestyle like playing tag with your kids or walking briskly with your dog for 10 minutes or more.

Hurdle: I have trouble staying disciplined.

Solution: Sharing your goal with a friend or family member and asking them to keep you accountable may help you keep your commitment. Setting small, realistic goals, checking your progress, and rewarding yourself when you reach your goal can also help. Research shows that if you can stick with an exercise routine or physical activity for at least 6 months, it's a good sign that you're on your way to making physical activity a regular habit.

Hurdle: The weather conditions where I live/during this time of year are not suitable for exercising outside.

Solution: You can take up yoga or Pilates as well as other indoor exercises that are easy to do with household items. The most important thing is to keep moving and walk whenever you can.

I'M JUST GETTING STARTED

If you are just getting started, start out slowly and add new physical activities little by little. After a few weeks or months, you can increase intensity by doing them longer and more often.

If you're not sure where to start, see the Activities and Levels of Exertion section for some examples of activities you could try.

CHOOSE ACTIVITIES THAT YOU ENJOY

Team up with a friend or join a class. Ask your family and friends to be active with you. Play games like volleyball or basketball.

Everyday activities can add up to an active lifestyle. You can:
- Go for a brisk walk around the neighborhood
- Ride a bicycle to work or just for fun
- Play outdoor games with your children

I'M DOING A LITTLE, BUT I'M READY TO GET MORE ACTIVE.

You may already be feeling the benefits of getting active, such as sleeping better or getting toned. Here are 2 ways to add more activity to your life.

Be active for longer each time you exercise. If you are walking 3 days a week for 30 minutes, try walking for an additional 10 minutes or more each day. Your goal is to meet your recommended amount of activity for your age and condition bracket, which is 2 hours and 30 minutes a week of moderate level activity including strength training for adults. (See the How Much Exercise Do I Need for My Age section).

Be active more often. If you are riding your bike to work 2 days a week, try doing it 4 days a week.

FIND TIME IN YOUR SCHEDULE
Planning time to exercise is one of the best ways to make sure that it happens. Many of those who say that they put it on their calendar for the week report that it would not have happened otherwise.

Look at your schedule for the week. Find a few 30-minute time periods you can use for more physical activity. Put them on your calendar. Try these ways to build more active time into your busy week.

Help your family move more each day and have fun with it. Think about what your family can do to be active together. Here are some ideas.[6]

Make Time
- Identify free times. Keep track of your daily activities for one week. Pick two 30-minute time slots that you could use for family activity time.

- Add physical activity to your daily routine. For example, walk or ride your bike to work or a friend's house, walk the dog with your children, or park farther away from your destination.

- Try to walk, jog, or swim during your lunch hour, or take fitness breaks instead of coffee breaks. Try doing something active with your family after dinner or on weekends.

Getting Started

- Find activities that require little time. Try walking, jogging, or stair climbing.

Bring Others Into It
- Ask friends and family to support your efforts.

- Invite them to be active with you.

- Set up a party or other social event with activities that get people moving, like having a jump rope contest.

- Exercise with friends.

- Play with your kids or ask them to join you for an exercise routine or fitness game.

- Develop new friendships with physically active people. Join a group such as the YMCA or a hiking club.

Energize Yourself
- Plan to be active at those times in the day or week when you feel you have a lot of energy.

- Convince yourself that if you give it a chance, physical activity will increase your energy level; then try it.

Stay Motivated
- Plan ahead. Make physical activity a regular part of your family's schedule. Write it on a family activity calendar.

- Join an exercise group or class.

- Pick activities requiring no new skills, such as walking or climbing stairs.

- Exercise with friends who are at the same skill level as you are. Create opportunities for your children to be active with friends.

Build New Skills
- Find a friend who can teach you new skills.

- Take a class to develop new skills and enroll your children in classes too, such as swimming, or tennis.

Use Available Resources
- Select activities that don't require costly sports gear, such as walking, jogging, jumping rope, or doing push-ups.

- Identify cheap, local resources in your area, such as programs through your community center, park or recreation group, or worksite.

Make the Most of All Conditions
- Develop a set of activities for you and your family that are always available regardless of weather, such as indoor cycling, indoor swimming, stair climbing, rope skipping, mall walking, and active games that you can play indoors.

- When the weather is nice, try outdoor swimming, jogging, walking, or tennis.

I'M ALREADY PHYSICALLY ACTIVE, AND I WANT TO KEEP IT UP.

Take Action: Challenge Yourself
If you are already active for 2 hours and 30 minutes each week, you can get even more health benefits by stepping up your routine.

Do More Vigorous Activities
In general, 15 minutes of vigorous activity has the same benefits as 30 minutes of moderate activity. Try jogging for 15 minutes instead of walking for 30 minutes.

Getting Started

EXAMPLE 1: Moderate Intensity Activity + Muscle Strengthening Activity

SUN	MON	TUE	WED	THU	FRI	SAT
30 Minute Brisk Walk	30 Minute Brisk Walk	30 Minute Brisk Walk	Weight Training	30 Minute Brisk Walk	30 Minute Brisk Walk	Weight Training

TOTAL: 150 minutes moderate-intensity aerobic activity + 2 days muscle-strengthening activity

EXAMPLE 2: Vigorous Intensity Activity + Muscle Strengthening Activity

SUN	MON	TUE	WED	THU	FRI	SAT
✗	25 Minute Jog	✗	25 Minute Jog + Weight Training	✗	Weight Training	25 Minute Jog

TOTAL: 75 minutes vigorous-intensity aerobic activity + 2 days muscle-strengthening activity

EXAMPLE 3: Mix of Moderate & Vigorous Intensity Activity + Muscle Strengthening Activity

SUN	MON	TUE	WED	THU	FRI	SAT
30 Minute Brisk Walk	15 Minute Jog	Weight Training	30 Minute Brisk Walk	Weight Training	15 Minute Jog	30 Minute Brisk Walk

TOTAL: The equivalent of 150 minutes of moderate-intensity aerobic activity + 2 days muscle-strengthening activity

Mix It Up

Mix vigorous activities with moderate ones. Try joining a fitness group or gym class. Don't forget to do muscle-strengthening activities 2 days a week.

Challenge Yourself

If you're thinking, "How can I meet the guidelines each week?" don't worry. There are a lot of ways to get the physical activity you need! You'll be surprised by the variety of activities from which you can choose. To meet the guidelines for aerobic activity, almost anything counts, as long as it's done at a moderate or vigorous intensity for at least 10 minutes at a time.

Stick With It

By picking physical activities you enjoy and that match your abilities, it will help ensure that you stick with them. If you're not sure where to start, here are some examples *(see page 149)*. If you're doing a little, but are ready to get more active, plan the time in your schedule to get more exercise.

"Nothing can substitute for just plain hard work. I had to put in the time to get back. And it was a grind. It meant training and sweating every day. But I was completely committed to working out to prove to myself that I still could do it."
- Andre Agassi

"Strength does not come from winning. Your struggles develop your strengths. When you go through hardships and decide not to surrender, that is strength."
- Arnold Schwarzenegger

"If you always put limits on everything you do, physical or anything else, it will spread into your work and into your life. There are no limits. There are only plateaus; and you must not stay there, you must go beyond them."
- Bruce Lee

"I'm not telling you it's going to be easy, I'm telling you it's going to be worth it."
- Art Williams

Chapter Eight
GETTING ACTIVE

EVERYDAY EXERCISE FOR THE WHOLE FAMILY[6]

Small steps that get your family to move more can help all of you maintain a healthy weight. Choose a different tip each week for you and your family to try. See if you or they can add to the list. Here are a few:

- Walk Whenever Possible
- Walk instead of drive whenever you can
- Walk your children to school
- Take the stairs instead of the escalator or elevator
- Take a family walk after dinner
- Replace a Sunday drive with a Sunday walk
- Go for a half-hour walk instead of watching TV
- Get off the bus a stop early and walk
- Park farther from the store and walk

- Make a Saturday morning walk a family habit
- Walk briskly in the mall
- Take the dog on longer walks
- Go up hills instead of around them

Move More in Your Home
- Garden, or make home repairs
- Do yard work. Get your children to help rake, weed, or plant
- Work around the house. Ask your children to help with active chores
- Wash the car by hand
- Use a snow shovel instead of a snow blower

Live Actively
- Join an exercise group, and enroll your children in community sports teams or lessons
- Have a sit-up competition with your kids
- Pace the sidelines at kids' athletic games
- Choose an activity that fits into your daily life/lives
- Use an exercise video if the weather is bad
- Avoid labor-saving devices, such as a remote control or electric mixers
- Play with your kids at least 30 minutes a day
- Explore new physical activities and sports
- Give yourself a gold star with non-food related rewards, such as a family day at the park, lake, or zoo
- Swim with your kids
- Make time for a half-day family activity each weekend, such as a family walk, bike ride, or volleyball game. Ask your kids which activity they most want to do.
- Play catch or soccer with your kids or organize a neighborhood game
- Plan an active family vacation or a weekend outing

- Play a backyard game such as freeze tag or Frisbee
- Buy a set of hand weights and play a round of Simon Says with your kids. (They run around without weights, you run around with weights; both getting exercise!)
- Take a nature hike to collect leaves and rocks to make a collage
- In the winter - Have a snowball fight, go ice skating or sledding
- Walk or bike to the local library to borrow a book

HELPING YOUR CHILDREN STAY FIT

If you want to help your children engage in more activity apart from exercising as a family, here are some tips. Parents can be a role model for their kids by leading a healthy lifestyle and by rewarding them for making healthy choices.

Eatright.org recommends planning time in your children's schedule to engage in 60 minutes of physical activity each day. These 60 minutes can accumulate with shorter periods throughout the day, but should be for at least 10 minutes at a time.

- Organize your family room or living room for more activity

- Set up a backyard net for badminton or other net-ball sports

- Encourage kids to participate in active chores such as light housework, raking leaves, sweeping the walks, or cleaning the garage. Make the chores fun to do — sing while doing them— and do the chores with them.

- Encourage fun, physical activity during kids' free time. The next time your kids say, "I'm bored," offer to shoot hoops or play catch.

- Enroll your kids in organized activities. These are a great way for kids to get fit. Encourage them to participate in a variety of activities such as soccer, swimming, or basketball.

STRETCHING

Stretching activities can be invigorating for your muscles and have proven to be a wonderful de-stressor. It is best to do the stretching after your muscles have warmed up to prevent straining them and causing an injury. It is important to do a warm-up with strength training to prevent injury. A cool-down routine is also vital to strength training and vigorous exercise like cardio work, to help repair muscles and prevent knots and cramps that could also lead to injury.

WARMUP[3]

5-minute Walk

To get your muscles warm and loose for strength training, walk for 5 to 10 minutes outside if weather permits, or inside around the house or on a treadmill if you have one. Walking will help direct needed blood flow to your muscles and prepare your body for exercise. Warming up is essential for preventing injury as well as gaining maximal benefit from the exercise, because loose, warm muscles will respond better to the challenge of lifting weights.

If you have another piece of aerobic exercise equipment available to you, such as a bike, rowing machine, or stair stepper, this will serve as an adequate warm up as well.

COOL DOWN[3]

Quadriceps Stretch

This excellent stretch should be a regular part of your cool down. Strength training exercises such as squats, step-ups, and knee extensions focus on strengthening the quadriceps muscles. This stretch will help these muscles relax and make them more flexible.

Getting Active

1. Stand next to a counter or sturdy chair with your feet about shoulder-width apart and your knees straight, but not locked.

2. With your left hand, hold the chair or counter for balance. Bend your right leg back and grasp your right ankle with your right hand until your thigh is perpendicular to the ground. Make sure you stand up straight—don't lean forward. (If you can't grasp your ankle in your hand, just keep your leg as close to perpendicular as possible and hold the bend, or place your foot on the seat of a chair.) You should feel a stretch in the front of the thigh.

3. Hold the stretch for a slow count of 20 to 30 seconds, breathing throughout.

4. Release your right ankle and repeat with the other leg.

Make sure you:
- Breathe throughout the stretch, concentrating on relaxing.
- Stand up straight and look straight ahead.
- Don't lock your supporting knee.

Hamstring/Calf Stretch
If touching your toes with straight legs seems an impossible task, you're not alone. Many people have tight hamstring and calf muscles in the back of the leg.

This stretch will give these muscles more flexibility and make it easier for you to bend over.

1. Sit forward in a chair with your knees bent and feet flat on the floor.

2. Extend your right leg in front of you, placing your right heel on the floor, and keeping your ankle relaxed. Don't lock your knee. Slowly lean forward at the hips, bending toward your

right toes, trying to keep your back straight.

3. Hold the stretch for a slow count of 20 to 30, breathing throughout.

4. Sit up straight again and flex your right ankle so that your toes are pointing up toward the ceiling. Again, lean forward at the hips, bending toward your right toes and hold the stretch for a slow count of 20 to 30, breathing throughout.

5. Release the stretch and repeat with your left leg.

Note: You should feel the first part of this stretch in the back of the upper leg and the second part in the calf.

Make sure you:
- Breathe throughout the stretch, concentrating on relaxing.
- Keep your back straight and head lifted as you lean forward toward your toes.
- Don't push the stretch too far—it shouldn't be painful.

Chest and Arm Stretch

This simple reaching stretch will improve the flexibility in your arms and chest and the front of your shoulders.

1. Stand with your arms at your sides and your feet about shoulder-width apart.

2. Extend both arms behind your back and clasp your hands together, if possible, retracting your shoulders.

3. Hold the stretch for a slow count of 20 to 30, breathing throughout.

4. Release the stretch and repeat.

Make sure you:
- Breathe throughout the stretch.
- Keep your back straight and look straight ahead.

Neck, Upper Back, and Shoulder Stretch

This easy stretch targets another group of muscles particularly vulnerable to tension and stress—the neck, back, and shoulders. Do it often—after strength training, and during any activity that makes you feel stiff, such as sitting at a desk or a computer. You'll find it rejuvenating.

1. Stand with your feet shoulder-width apart, your knees straight but not locked, and your hands clasped in front of you.

2. Rotate your hands so that your palms are facing the ground; then raise your arms to about chest height.

3. Gently press your palms away from your body. You should feel a stretch in your neck and upper back and along your shoulders.

4. Hold the stretch for a slow count of 20 to 30, breathing throughout.

5. Release the stretch and repeat.

Make sure you:
- Breathe throughout the stretch.
- Don't curve or arch your back.

STRENGTH TRAINING FOR ALL LEVELS[18]

Physical and mental health benefits that can be achieved through resistance training include:
- Improved muscle strength and tone – to protect your joints from injury. It also helps you maintain flexibility and balance and helps you remain independent as you age

- Weight management and increased muscle-to-fat ratio – as you gain muscle, your body burns more calories when at rest
- Greater stamina – as you grow stronger, you won't tire as easily
- Prevention or control of chronic conditions such as diabetes, heart disease, arthritis, back pain, depression, and obesity
- Pain management
- Improved mobility and balance
- Improved posture
- Decreased risk of injury
- Increased bone density and strength and reduced risk of osteoporosis
- Improved sense of well-being – resistance training may boost your self-confidence, improve your body image, and lighten your mood
- A better night's sleep and avoidance of insomnia
- Increased self-esteem
- Enhanced performance of everyday tasks.

Muscle-Strengthening Activities[3]

As an adult, besides aerobic activity, you need to do things to make your muscles stronger at least 2 days a week.

To provide real health benefits, muscle-strengthening activities need to be done to the point where it's hard for you to do another repetition without help. A repetition is one complete movement of an activity, such as lifting a weight or doing one sit-up. Try to do 8—12 repetitions per activity that count as 1 set. Try to do at least 1 set of muscle-strengthening activities, but to gain even more benefits, do 2 or 3 sets.

There are many ways you can strengthen your muscles, whether it's at home or at the gym. The activities you choose should work all the major muscle groups of your body (legs, hips, back, chest, abdomen, shoulders, and arms). You may want to try:

- Lifting weights
- Working with resistance bands
- Doing exercises that use your body weight for resistance (push-ups, sit ups)
- Heavy gardening (digging, shoveling)

LOW INTENSITY STRENGTH TRAINING

The CDC recommends the following strength training program for beginners and older adults who want to build strength, maintain bone density, and reduce the risk of falling. It will also improve balance, coordination, and mobility, and help you maintain independence in performing the activities of daily life. It is safe and recommended for all ages. Whatever your age, medical condition, or current level of activity, you are likely a perfect candidate for this gentle but powerful regimen of strengthening exercises.

Growing Strong Program - Stage 1

The following four exercises comprise Stage 1 of the Growing Stronger Program. When you've been doing the exercises of this stage for at least two weeks, or if you are relatively fit right now, you can add the exercises in Stage 2. Remember always to do the warm-up and cool-down as part of each exercise session.

- Squats
- Wall Pushups
- Toe Stands
- Finger Marching

Squats

A great exercise for strengthening hips, thighs, and buttocks. Before long, you'll find that walking, jogging, and climbing stairs are a snap! *Use a chair for safety.*

1. In front of a sturdy, armless chair, stand with feet slightly more than shoulder-width apart. Extend your arms out so they are parallel to the ground and lean forward a little at the hips.

2. Making sure that your knees NEVER come forward past your toes, lower yourself in a slow, controlled motion to a count of four, until you reach a near-sitting position.

3. Pause. Then, to a count of two, slowly rise back up to a standing position. Keep your knees over your ankles and your back straight.

4. Repeat 10 times for one set. Rest for one to two minutes. Then complete a second set of 10 repetitions.

Note 1: If this exercise is too difficult, start off by using your hands for assistance. If you are unable to go all the way down, place a couple of pillows on the chair or only squat down four to six inches.

Note 2: Placing more weight on your heels than on the balls or toes of your feet can help keep your knees from moving forward past your toes. It will also cause you to use the muscles of your hips more during the rise to a standing position.

Make sure you:
- Don't sit down too quickly.
- Don't lean your weight too far forward or onto your toes when standing up.

Wall Pushups

This exercise is a modified version of the push-up you may have done years ago in physical education classes. It is less challenging than a classic push-up and won't require you to get down on the floor—but it will help to strengthen your arms, shoulders, and chest.

1. Find a wall that is clear of any objects—wall hangings, windows, etc. Stand a little farther than arm's length from the wall.

2. Facing the wall, lean your body forward and place your palms flat against the wall at about shoulder height and shoulder-width apart.

3. To a count of four, bend your elbows as you lower your upper body toward the wall in a slow, controlled motion, keeping your feet planted.

4. Pause. Then, to a count of two, slowly push yourself back until your arms are straight—but don't lock your elbows.

5. Repeat 10 times for one set. Rest for one to two minutes. Then complete a second set of 10 repetitions.

Make sure you:
- Don't round or arch your back.

Toe Stands

If a walk in the park no longer seems easy or enjoyable, the "toe stand" exercise is for you! A good way to strengthen your calves and ankles and restore stability and balance, it will help make that stroll in the park fun and relaxing.

1. Near a counter or sturdy chair, stand with feet shoulder-width apart. Use the chair or counter for balance.

2. To a count of four, slowly push up as far as you can onto the balls of your feet and hold for two to four seconds.

3. Then, to a count of four, slowly lower your heels back to the floor.

4. Repeat 10 times for one set. Rest for one to two minutes. Then complete a second set of 10 repetitions.

Make sure you:
- Don't lean on the counter or chair—use them for balance only.
- Breathe regularly throughout the exercise.

Finger Marching

In this exercise you'll let your fingers, hands, and arms do the walking. This will help strengthen your upper body and your grip, and increase the flexibility of your arms, back, and shoulders.

1. Stand, or sit forward in an armless chair, with feet on the floor, shoulder-width apart.

2. Movement 1: Imagine there is a wall directly in front of you. Slowly walk your fingers up the wall until your arms are above your head. Hold them overhead while wiggling your fingers for about 10 seconds and then slowly walk them back down.

3. Movement 2: Next, try to touch your two hands behind your back. If you can, reach for the opposite elbow with each hand—or get as close as you can. Hold the position for about 10 seconds, feeling a stretch in the back, arms, and chest.

4. Movement 3: Release your arms and finger-weave your hands in front of your body. Raise your arms so that they're parallel to the ground, with your palms facing the imaginary wall. Sit or stand up straight, but curl your shoulders forward. You should feel the stretch in your wrist and upper back. Hold the position for about 10 seconds.

5. Repeat this three-part exercise three times.

Growing Strong Program - Stage 2

When you've been doing the exercises from Stage 1 for at least two weeks, OR if you are relatively fit right now, you can add these Stage 2 exercises. When you've been doing the exercises from Stages 1 and 2 for at least six weeks, you can add the exercises in Stage 3. Remember always to do the warm-up and cool-down as part of each exercise session.

- Biceps Curl
- Step Ups
- Overhead Press
- Hip Abduction

Biceps Curl

Does a gallon of milk feel a lot heavier than it used to? After a few weeks of doing the biceps curl, lifting that eight-pound jug will seem a cinch!

1. With a dumbbell in each hand, either stand, or sit in an armless chair with feet shoulder-width apart, arms at your sides, and palms facing your thighs.

2. To a count of two, slowly lift up the weights so that your forearms rotate and palms face in toward your shoulders while keeping your upper arms and elbows close to your side—as if you had a newspaper tucked under your arm. Keep your wrists straight, and dumbbells parallel to the floor.

3. Pause. Then, to a count of four, slowly lower the dumbbells back toward your thighs, rotating your forearms so that your arms are again at your sides, with palms facing your thighs.

4. Repeat 10 times for one set. Rest for one to two minutes. Then complete a second set of 10 repetitions.

Make sure you:
- Don't let your elbows move away from the sides of your body.
- Keep your wrists straight.

Step Ups

This is a great strengthening exercise that requires only a set of stairs, but don't let its simplicity fool you. Step-ups will improve your balance and build strength in your legs, hips, and buttocks.

1. Stand alongside the handrail at the bottom of a staircase. With your feet flat and toes facing forward, put your right foot on the first step.

2. Holding the handrail for balance, to a count of two, straighten your right leg to lift up your left leg slowly until it reaches the first step. As you're lifting yourself up, make sure that your right knee stays straight and does not move forward past your ankle. Let your left foot tap the first step near your right foot.

3. Pause. Then, using your right leg to support your weight, to a count of four, slowly lower your left foot back to the floor.

4. Repeat 10 times with the right leg and 10 times with the left leg for one set. Rest for one to two minutes. Then complete a second set of 10 repetitions with each leg.

Make sure you:

- Don't let your back leg do the work.

- Don't let momentum do the work.

- Press your weight through the heel rather than ball or toes of your front leg as you lift.

Overhead Press

This useful exercise targets several muscles in the arms, upper back, and shoulders. It can also help firm the back of your upper arms and make reaching for objects in high cupboards easier.

1. Stand or sit in an armless chair with feet shoulder-width apart. With a dumbbell in each hand, raise your hands, palms facing forward, until the dumbbells are level with your shoulders and parallel to the floor.

2. To a count of two, slowly push the dumbbells up over your head until your arms are fully extended—but don't lock your elbows.

3. Pause. Then, to a count of four, slowly lower the dumbbells back to shoulder level, bringing your elbows down close to your sides.

4. Repeat 10 times for one set. Rest for one to two minutes. Then complete a second set of 10 repetitions.

Make sure you:
- Keep your wrists straight.
- Don't lock your elbows.
- Don't let the dumbbells move too far in front of, or behind, your body.
- Breathe throughout the exercise.

Hip Abduction

By targeting the muscles of the hips, thighs, and buttocks, this exercise strengthens your hipbones, which may be especially vulnerable to fracture as you age.

1. Stand behind a sturdy chair, with feet slightly apart and toes facing forward. Keep your legs straight, but do not lock your knees.

2. To a count of two, slowly lift your right leg out to the side. Keep your left leg straight—but again, do not lock your knee.

3. Pause. Then, to a count of four, slowly lower your right foot back to the ground.

4. Repeat 10 times with the right leg and 10 times with the left leg for one set. Rest for one to two minutes. Then complete a second set of 10 repetitions with each leg.

Make sure you:
- Don't lock your knee on the supporting leg.
- Keep your toes facing forward throughout the move.
- Don't lean to the side when you lift your leg.

To increase the difficulty of this exercise, you may add ankle weights.

Growing Strong Program - Stage 3
When you've been doing the exercises from Stage 1 and Stage 2 for at least six weeks, you can add these Stage 3 exercises. Remember to always do the warm-up and cool-down as part of each exercise session:

- Knee Extension
- Knee Curl
- Pelvic Tilt
- Floor Back Extension

Knee Extension
By targeting the quadriceps muscles in the front of the thigh (which play a primary role in bending and straightening the leg), this exercise strengthens weak knees and reduces the symptoms of arthritis of the knee. It is important to do this exercise in conjunction with Exercise 10, the "knee curl," as the muscles targeted in these two exercises—the front thigh muscles and the hamstrings—work together when you walk, stand, and climb.

1. Put on your ankle weights.

2. In a sturdy, armless chair, sit all the way back, so that your feet

barely touch the ground; this will allow for easier movement throughout the exercise. If your chair is too low, add a rolled-up towel under your knees. Your feet should be shoulder-width apart, and your arms should rest at your sides or on your thighs.

3. With your toes pointing forward and your foot flexed, to a count of two, slowly lift your right leg, extending your leg until your knee is straight.

4. Pause. Then, to a count of four, slowly lower your foot back to the ground.

5. Repeat 10 times with the right leg and 10 times with the left leg for one set. Rest for a minute or two. Then complete a second set of 10 repetitions with each leg.

Make sure you:

- Keep your ankle flexed throughout the move.

Knee Curl

This is an excellent exercise for strengthening the muscles of the back of the upper leg, known as the hamstrings. When done in conjunction with the knee extension, it makes walking and climbing easier.

1. Put on your ankle weights.

2. Stand behind a sturdy chair, with feet shoulder-width apart and facing forward.

3. Keeping your foot flexed, to a count of two, slowly bend your right leg, bringing your heel up toward your buttocks.

4. Pause. Then, to a count of four, slowly lower your foot back to the ground.

5. Repeat 10 times with your right leg and 10 times with your left leg for one set. Rest for a minute or two. Then complete a second set of 10 repetitions with each leg.

Make sure you:
- Keep the thigh of the bending leg in line with the supporting leg at all times.
- Keep the foot on the bending leg flexed throughout the move.

Pelvic Tilt

This exercise improves posture and tightens the muscles in your abdomen and buttocks. Do this exercise in conjunction with the floor back extension to strengthen your midsection. (You should not have the ankle weights on during this exercise.)

1. On the floor or on a firm mattress, lie flat on your back with your knees bent, feet flat and arms at your sides, palms facing the ground.

2. To a count of two, slowly roll your pelvis so that your hips and lower back are off the floor, while your upper back and shoulders remain in place.

3. Pause. Then, to a count of four, slowly lower your pelvis all the way down.

4. Repeat 10 times for one set. Rest for a minute or two. Then complete a second set of 10 repetitions.

Make sure you:
- Breathe throughout the exercise.
- Don't lift your upper back or shoulders off the ground.

Floor Back Extension

If you suffer from lower back pain, weak abdominal muscles may be to blame. The floor back extension, done in conjunction with the pelvic tilt, will strengthen these muscles and ease back pain.

1. Lie on the floor facedown, with two pillows under your hips. Extend your arms straight overhead on the floor.

2. To a count of two, slowly lift your right arm and left leg off the floor, keeping them at the same level.

3. Pause. Then, to a count of four, slowly lower your arm and leg back to the floor.

4. Repeat 10 times for one set, and then switch to left arm with right leg for another 10 repetitions.

5. Rest for a minute or two. Then complete a second set of 10 repetitions.

Make sure you:
- Keep your head, neck, and back in a straight line.

MODERATE - VIGOROUS INTENSITY **STRENGTH TRAINING**

Complete warm-up and cool-down activities before strength training.

Beginners Strength Training Plan[13]

- 20 body weight squats
- 10 push ups
- 20 walking lunges
- 10 dumbbell rows (using a gallon milk jug)
- 15 second plank
- 30 jumping jacks

For adults, do this routine 2-3 times a week. Do not do it two days in a row, however, as muscle is built when you're resting. See the How Much Exercise Do I Need? chapter for a recommended plan.

Remember, with strength training, it is important to eat properly as well. Protein will help to build muscle, and natural, whole foods will help you stay lean. Steve Kamb, fitness trainer and nutrition author of nerdfitness.com says, "Your diet is at least 80% of your success or failure (in strength training)."

Body Weight Squats
Think of this activity as sitting back onto a chair. If you can sit down onto a chair, and then stand immediately back up without having to lean forward, you are doing it right.

Form and starting position:

- Stand with your feet slightly wider than your hips. Your toes should be pointed slightly outward.

- Look straight ahead, picking a spot in front of you.

- You can put your arms straight out in front of you, parallel to the ground, or behind your head if you like.

- Keep your spine in a neutral position, not rounding it out or pushing it in.

- Your weight should be on the heels and balls of your feet.

- Keep your whole body tight the entire time.

Squat down:
Move into a sitting position. Begin the movement by flexing your knees and hips; moving back with your hips. It's important that you start with moving your hips back, and not by bending your knees. Your knees should not extend forward past your feet. Keep your back straight, your neutral spine, and your

chest and shoulders up. Keep looking straight ahead at that spot on the wall.

Return to position
Squat down until your hip joint is lower than your knees if you are able, and quickly reverse the motion until you return to the starting position. As you squat, keep your head and chest up and push your knees out.

If you can't do it properly at first, you can put your hand onto a support to help you keep your balance.

Push Ups[12]

Begin on your hands and knees
Place your hands firmly on the floor, directly under shoulders. Walk your feet back until you are on your hands and toes, with your legs and back in a straight line.

Lower your body
Begin to lower your body—keeping your back flat and eyes focused about three feet in front of you until your chest grazes the floor. Don't let your hips drop or your back arch at any point during the move; your body should remain in a straight line from head to toe. Draw shoulder blades back and down, keeping elbows tucked close to your body (don't "T" your arms).

Push back up
Keeping your core engaged, exhale as you push back to the starting position.

Common Push-Up Mistakes
- Letting your lower back sag or arch

- Forgetting to breathe - Concentrating on form and reps can make it easy to forget one of the most important parts of working out: breathing. Inhale on the way down and exhale on the way up.

- Flaring your arms - Letting your arms pop out to 90 degrees can be hard on the shoulders. Instead of forming a "T" with the arms and body, keep your elbows tucked close, at about a 20- to 40-degree angle to your torso.

- Cheating Yourself - Make sure each push-up reaches a full range of motion by getting your chest as close to the floor as comfortable, then fully extending your elbows at the top.

- Straining Your Neck - You can fix this by picking a point on the floor a few feet in front of you to focus on.

Walking Lunges[12]

1. Begin by standing with your feet shoulder-width apart and your hands on your hips.

2. Step forward with one leg, flexing the knees to drop your hips. Descend until your rear knee nearly touches the ground. Your posture should remain upright, and your front knee should stay above the front foot.

3. Drive through the heel of your lead foot and extend both knees to raise yourself back up.

4. Step forward with your rear foot, repeating the lunge on the opposite leg.

If you can't do it properly at first, you can put your hand on a support to help you keep your balance.

Dumbbell Rows[15]

Variation: You can replace dumbbells with a milk jug or anything that is heavy enough for you. You should be able to lift the weight 10 times in a row.

1. Choose a flat bench and place a dumbbell on each side of it.

2. Place the right knee on top of the end of the bench, bend your torso forward from the waist until your upper body is parallel to the floor, and place your right hand on the other end of the bench for support.

3. Use the left hand to pick up the dumbbell on the floor and hold the weight while keeping your lower back straight. The palm of the hand should be facing your torso. This will be your starting position.

4. Pull the resistance straight up to the side of your chest, keeping your upper arm close to your side and keeping the torso stationary. Breathe out as you perform this step. Tip: Concentrate on squeezing the back muscles once you reach the full contracted position. Also, make sure that the force is performed with the back muscles and not the arms. Finally, the upper torso should remain stationary, and only the arms should move. The forearms should do no other work except for holding the dumbbell; therefore do not try to pull the dumbbell up using the forearms.

5. Lower the resistance straight down to the starting position. Breathe in as you perform this step.

6. Repeat the movement for the specified amount of repetitions.

7. Switch sides and repeat with the other arm.

Planks[12]
Standard Plank
1. Plant the hands directly under the shoulders (slightly wider than shoulder-width apart) like you're about to do a push-up.

2. Ground the toes on the floor and squeeze the glutes to stabilize the body. Your legs should be working in the move too. Be careful not to lock or hyperextend your knees.

3. Neutralize the neck and spine by looking at a spot on the floor about a foot beyond the hands. Your head should be in line with your back.

4. Hold the position for 20 seconds. As you get more comfortable with the move, hold your plank for as long as possible without compromising form or breathing.

Plank Variations
Forearm Plank
The forearm plank is one of the most common ways to do a plank and is slightly easier than the standard version.

1. Place the forearms on the ground with the elbows aligned below the shoulders, and arms parallel to the body at about shoulder-width distance. If flat palms bother your wrists, clasp your hands together.

Knee Plank
The knee plank is a step easier than the forearm plank, making it great for beginners because it allows them to concentrate on form. By resting the knees on the ground, there's less stress on the lower back.

1. Rest your knees on a rolled up mat or towel if they feel uncomfortable on the floor.

Jumping Jacks
1. Stand with your feet together and your hands down by your side.

2. In one motion jump your feet out to the side and raise your arms above your head.

3. Immediately reverse that motion by jumping back to the starting position.

Getting Active

RUNNING

Running Tips for Beginners[10]

One of the easiest forms of cardio exercise that people adopt is running, because it doesn't require any equipment besides your running shoes. You can do it just about anywhere, and it burns more calories than almost any other mainstream exercise.

Regular running can reduce your risk of chronic illnesses such as heart disease, type 2 diabetes, and stroke. It can also boost your mood and help keep your weight under control. Running is an ideal choice for many people.

The National Health Service (NHS) in the UK gives a guide to make running a safe and enjoyable experience for beginners, and to provide you with tips on how to stay motivated.

Before you start

For those who are recovering from an injury, have a chronic illness, or feel especially out of shape, it is recommended to see your doctor before running.

Running can be an exhausting and discouraging sport for those who are not used to it; however, if you start slowly and work your way up to pace it can be very enjoyable! If you have not been active for a while, to begin with a walking routine can be a great start.

A good pair of shoes can help prevent injury. Invest in shoes that are designed for running, which are better padded than a walking shoe. Most workers at athletic stores can help you find the best fit for your foot and arch. It's advisable to replace running shoes every 300 miles, as a shoe's shock absorbers weaken over time, increasing your risk of injury.

To Start Running

1. Start each run with a gentle warm-up of at least five minutes.

This can include quick walking, marching on the spot, knee lifts, side stepping, and climbing stairs for anywhere from 530 minutes.

2. Your running form should include running with your arms and shoulders relaxed and elbows bent. Keep an upright posture and a smooth stride, striking the ground with the middle of your foot.

3. Run at a pace that feels comfortable to you. You don't have to run at maximum effort, especially if you are aiming at endurance running. Running slower will help you to run longer. As you progress, you can add speed training if you like.

4. The NHS recommends that once you can walk for 30 minutes easily, include some running intervals of one to two minutes at a speed that feels comfortable. As time goes on, make the running intervals longer, until you're running for 30 minutes continuously.

5. After your run, give yourself a few moments to cool down and bring your heartbeat back to normal. You can do this by walking, followed by gently stretching your leg muscles after each run. Refrain from sitting down or remaining dormant right after a run, as muscles can tighten and injure.

6. To maintain your progress, it is recommended that you run at least twice a week. Consistency is key in running, as you will see yourself improve and be able to add distance and time to your runs each week.

KEEPING YOURSELF MOTIVATED
Set yourself a goal
Whatever your level, setting goals is a great way to stay motivated. Signing up for a race like a 5K could be the perfect inspiration to help you develop a routine of running, and most likely you will be

hooked afterward. The reward of finishing a race is exhilarating.

Run with a friend
It's a big help to have someone at about the same level of ability as yourself to run with. You'll encourage each other when you don't feel like running. The accountability of someone waiting on you or needing you to help them with their fitness will motivate you.

Add variety
Keep your running interesting by mixing it up. Running the same route over and over again can become boring. Vary your distances and routes.

RUNNER'S WORLD GIVES SOME ADVICE FROM EXPERIENCED RUNNERS:

- Invest in the right pair of running shoes (You can ask your local athletic store to help you find the best fit for your foot and arch).

- Go for distance rather than time - Run at the pace you're comfortable with and don't worry about others. Be patient with yourself and slowly build up your speed.

- Mix in cross training to supplement your running
    Cross training, working muscles other than those used while running, is important for supporting your runs. Try swimming, canoeing, strength training, or bicycling.

- Remember to rest
    Running every day is hard on the muscles; they need time to repair. Running every day will actually slow down your progress instead of building it. You can choose to cross train on rest days if you like.

- Join a running group
    Although running on your own is necessary as a runner, it can get lonely and boring. Running with a group can help challenge you and re-motivate you.

- Make running a habit, even if that means carving out a few minutes to do so every day.
    Running consistently is much better for your endurance than long runs spaced far apart.

- Build mileage gradually

- Don't dread taking walk breaks
    Walking and running intervals have been proven to build strength and endurance to benefit your running.

- Keep a training log
    Many have found a running log to be very helpful in their journey to becoming a better runner. Keep track of when and how long you ran, the weather conditions, what you ate before and after, and how you felt during the run. This will help you to see ways to improve the quality of your run and set yourself up for success.

- Set small, achievable goals
    Break down your aspirations into daily, weekly, and monthly goals.

- Remember that you are a runner
    One of the biggest challenges new runners face is fearing that they aren't really a "runner." Whenever you're in doubt, remember these wise words from Chief Running World Officer Bart Yasso: "I often hear someone say, "I'm not a real runner." We are all runners, some just run faster than others. I never met a fake runner."

TIPS FROM EXPERIENCED RUNNERS[11]

For those who already love running but need some advice for increasing speed or the quality of their runs, here are some tips. Experienced runners should be running 3 or more days a week, but still taking at least one day a week to rest and recover.

Increase Mileage - Try boosting your weekly mileage by about 20 percent over the course of 4 to 6 weeks. The extra mileage shouldn't be difficult if you are running consistently. A typical training plan for those increasing their mileage for a race or goal usually includes running 3-4 days during the week with easy/short runs and then doing a longer run on the weekends. You should be able to add a mile to the long weekend run, and to one of the midweek runs each week, keeping the others short and easy.

Increase Speed - One of the best ways to increase speed is to break the routine of just "running" and add sprints and hill work. Speed work, done the proper way, has multiple benefits including injury prevention. Here is an example of hill sprints that you can do:

Hill Sprints[13]
- Start with 2 to 4 hill sprints lasting only eight seconds each.
- Run the first one at 95 percent maximum speed, while the rest are at 100 percent effort (running as fast as you possibly can).
- Find a very steep hill, one that you would normally avoid for regular hill repetitions.
- Take a full 1 to 2 minutes of walking recovery in between each one. Don't rush these.
- Run hill sprints after an easy or moderate run, 1 to 2 times per week
- Build to 6 to 8 reps that last 10 seconds each

OTHER EXERCISES YOU CAN DO AT HOME

Bath Towel

File this one under brilliant! Your bath towel can double as a nifty exercise band. Can't touch your toes? No worries, your towel can! A good old bathroom towel can provide you with valuable assistance to all your stretches in hard-to-reach areas, such as the seated hamstring stretch.

Sit on a pillow with your feet far apart, twist your body so that the middle of your chest is pointed toward the middle of the knee then put the towel around the arch of your foot and lean down, breathing gently. Hold for a minute then switch sides.

Chair

Do each exercise for 40 seconds and repeat four sets a few times a week.

- Toe taps: Standing near a chair (or stool), alternate tapping toes on the platform. By driving your knees up toward your chest and increasing your pace, you will increase the intensity. For more of a challenge, jump to switch your feet. To modify, use a lower step or stool and slow your pace.

- Triceps dip: Placing your hands on the edge of a chair or bench, lift your hips up and keep your shoulders over your hips; knees over ankles. To isolate your triceps, bend your elbows to a 90-degree angle then re-extend the arms. You can speed up the pace to increase the burn, or slow it down by lifting for two counts and lowering for two counts.

- Mountain climbers/knee tucks: Push into a straight-arm plank (upper push-up position). Place your feet on gliders, a towel or even socks on a hard floor; keep your shoulders over wrists and core engaged. Alternate drawing knees into the chest. For more of a challenge, draw both knees in simultaneously or pick up your pace with single legs. To modify or without a slick surface, you can take a mountain climber position by running the knees into the chest instead of sliding.

Wall
No matter how humble your abode, everyone's got at least one per room. So pick a wall and place your upper back against it. Lower yourself and sit down into a squat so that your legs are at a 90-degree angle and hold steady for 30 to 60 seconds. Keep your abs engaged as you hold the squat. Wall squats are an excellent way to tone your legs and your core at the same time!

Rice Bags
Those tasty rice bowl recipes you've been churning out for dinner lately may just do double duty for your health. Ricebag workouts don't have to be difficult. As an introductory move, start off slow by using bags of rice to stabilize your upper body when learning to squat. Or, try doing sit-stand-sit squats onto a couch holding a rice bag. The rice bag will stop you from using momentum instead of leg strength to get you off the couch- an excellent habit to build!

Book or Box
Talk about easy and effective! Push a book against the wall or find a sturdy box or crate to perform a step workout or elevated lunges. For the step workout, step one foot on the book or crate and then step the other foot onto the surface. Step one foot back on the floor and then the other. For elevated lunges, place one foot on the surface and perform a regular lunge. Alternate sides.

Large Bottle of Liquid Laundry Detergent
These are perfect to use for even the most complicated of kettlebell or free-weight moves. Keep it light by filling with water or make

it heavy by adding dirt and water to make it heavier. No laundry detergent? No problem. You can also use the gallon-sized plastic milk containers.

Decorative Pillow
Turns out, your killer sense of decor can help your cardio workouts as well. For hand-to-feet ball passes, lie on the floor with your arms extended over your head and place the pillow (or any kind of sports ball you may have) between your ankles. Keep your head, shoulders and back on the floor. Slowly raise your feet and your arms to meet above your torso, with arms and legs fully outstretched. Pass the ball or pillow from your ankles to your hands and lower legs and arms back to the floor. Repeat the action, passing the ball or pillow from your hands to your ankles. Continue passing back and forth for as many repetitions as possible.

Soup Cans
Use a two or three pound can of food for a quick arm blast! Genius. It's all about being creative. There are small weights like soup cans all around your home. Soup or bean cans are ideal if you are new to lifting weights but any canned food will work. Experiment with simple moves like bicep curls, hammer curls, overhead shoulder presses, and tricep kickbacks.

For the Love of Living

Chapter Nine
EXERCISING TO LOSE WEIGHT

Exercising is a great way to help you lose weight. In fact, combined with a healthy diet, it is the most effective way to lose weight and keep it off.

There are a lot of crash and fad diets advertised in today's market. You might have tried some of them and maybe even saw results. However, most people who lose weight from fad diets that restrict major food groups or involve fasting or diet pills, regain their starting weight and sometimes more. The reason is that these diets are not realistic or healthy for long-term weight management.

In reality, weight loss is a simple formula. Here we will discuss proven and healthy ways to lose weight.

1. Don't be in too much of a hurry – The main reason why people try fad diets is because they promise weight loss fast! They

involve limitations and fasting regimens that are hard and often unrealistic. Even if the diet can be adhered to long enough to lose some weight, it usually cannot be maintained long-term; the weight is regained and sometimes more is added. Remember, seeking a healthy lifestyle that works for you and that you can maintain long-term is the ultimate goal. Depending on your size, a healthy amount of weight to lose per week is 2-3 pounds.

2. Burn more calories than you eat - This is the simple formula to losing weight. So if you want to lose weight now, you'll have to eat less and exercise more. For instance, if you take in 1,000-1,200 calories a day and exercise for 20-40 minutes per day, you could lose 2-3 pounds in the first week, or more if you weigh more than 250 pounds. It is critical not to cut any more than 1,000-1,200 calories per day, as it is then counterproductive and dangerous.

3. Choose wholesome foods - As long as you eat fewer calories than you burn, you can eat whatever you want. However, choosing better foods will help your body to lose weight even faster. Here are some basic recommendations from Dawn Jackson Blatner, RD, author of Flexitarian Diet:

   - Eat vegetables to help you feel full

   - Drink plenty of water

   - Get tempting foods out of your home

   - Stay busy - you don't want to eat just because you're bored

   - Eat only from a plate, while seated at a table. Placing food on a plate will aid in portion control. Refrain from eating out of the bag or box or grazing in front of the 'fridge or pantry.

- Don't skip meals - this will cause blood sugar spikes, which will cause poor digestion of your next meal and actually cause you to gain weight.

- Keep a food journal - writing down everything you eat will help you to know how many calories you're eating and can help you stay on track.

4. Don't deprive yourself of foods you love- The reason why most fad diets don't work is that when you deprive yourself of foods that you love, you end up abandoning your diet and bingeing on those foods. As long as you are staying within your calorie intake, it is ok to eat foods that you crave, but be sure to portion them out and track them in your calorie count. There is quite a bit of research that shows that a taking a "cheat day" where you eat what you want one day a week, is helpful to maintain discipline. When you return to your diet the next day, it balances itself out.

5. Keep a food and exercise log – Since consuming fewer calories than you burn is the way to lose weight, the best way to ensure this is to keep track of what you eat and how much you exercise. Keeping track of what you eat will help to keep yourself accountable. Often the food you eat has more calories than you think, especially when snacking.

EXERCISES FOR INCREASED FAT BURNING

To lose weight, you will want to follow at least the recommended exercise amounts for your age group (How Much Exercise Do I Need? section). If you are an adult, that would mean exercising 35 times a week doing moderate to vigorous intensity workouts and strength training at least 2 times in between. WebMD says that according to studies, losing weight often requires an hour a day of moderate exercise.

Cardio exercise and strength training are the best exercises for burning fat. Cardio activity burns the most calories, as it keeps your heart rate up. To burn the most fat, try to break a sweat after you warm up and continue sweating for the entire hour. You will want to supplement cardio work with strength training because it will keep your metabolism up and give you the energy you need to exercise. Muscle tissue also burns more calories -- even when you're at rest.

Remember to pace yourself if you are a beginner. You may not be able to complete the full round of exercise at first.

INTERVAL TRAINING

For those who are working their way up to vigorous intensity work and for those who want a challenge, interval training is a good option. Interval training is training in which an athlete alternates between two activities, typically requiring different rates of speed, degrees of effort, etc. Interval training allows you to work harder without having to stay at an intense level for the whole duration of the workout. It is proven that the more you do it, the easier it becomes to burn more calories. You can try these workouts from builtlean.com:

To time yourself, you can watch a clock on the wall, use a countdown timer on a watch, or use a stopwatch.

100 Meter Walk-back Sprint
- Warm-up with stretches and a light jog. Then, on a track, sprint 100m as fast as you can and walk back to the start.
- Repeat 4-10x.

25 Minute Sprint
- Jog for 8 minutes
- Fast run for 4 minutes

- Sprint for 20 seconds
- Walk for 1 minute
- Sprint for 30 seconds
- Walk for 1 minute
- Sprint for 10 seconds
- Walk for 1 minute
- Jog for 5 minutes.
- Complete a fast run for 1 minute to the finish and then cool down by walking for 5-10 minutes at the end.

Countdown Jump Rope Workout
- For 2 minutes, complete as many jump rope revolutions as you can
- Rest 2 minutes
- For 1.5 minutes, complete as many jump rope revolutions as you can
- Rest For 1.5 minutes
- For 1 minute, complete as many jump rope revolutions as you can
- Rest for 1 minute
- For 30 seconds, complete as many jump rope revolutions as you can
- Rest for 3 minutes, then repeat 1-2x

This gives you an idea for interval training. You can vary the time and activity however you like.

For the Love of Living

Chapter Ten

TRACKING YOUR PROGRESS

Tracking your progress and logging the details of your exercise and diet can be one of the best ways to excel!

Log each exercise and note how you felt while doing it. You may also want to note what you ate before exercising to see how it affected your performance and energy.

- Log your calories for a couple of days to a few weeks in order to understand how many calories you are taking in, compared to what you are burning. You can find nutrition facts online or print a hard-copy of the National Institute of Health's fat and calorie counter here: *http://www.niddk.nih.gov/health-information/health-communication-programs/ndep/health-care-professionals/game-plan/small-steps/Documents/gp_fatcal.pdf*

- There are also many mobile applications like MyFitnessPal and LoseIt that will help you track your exercise, food, and weight loss goals.

- Take time to journal weekly after starting your exercise regimen. Note how you feel and how the week went. Doing this will help you to see how far you've come and know how to improve.

Use the following journal questions to help you track your progress for the first six weeks. If desired, continue using the same questions in a separate journal for the time beyond that.

Before starting

- What is your current activity level?

- How do you feel? What is your current energy level?

- How do you feel about starting exercising?

- What is your long-term goal?

- What is your goal for the next week?

Journal about any other thoughts and feelings you have at this point.

FREQUENTLY ASKED QUESTIONS

IS PHYSICAL ACTIVITY FOR EVERYONE?[2]
Yes! Physical activity is good for people of all ages and body types. Even if you feel out-of-shape or you haven't been active in a long time, you can find activities that will work for you. Seek the advice of your doctor if you have a current health condition that may limit you to certain exercises.

HOW LONG DO I NEED TO BE ACTIVE BEFORE I SEE RESULTS?
Once you start being physically active, you'll begin to see results in just a few weeks. You may feel stronger and more energetic than before. You may notice that you can do things more easily, faster, or for longer than before. As you become more fit, you may need to make your activities more challenging to see additional results. As your body gets used to a level of exercise, you'll need to vary your exercise or do more in order to see further progress as well.

I HAVE A MEDICAL CONDITION (SUCH AS ARTHRITIS, HIGH BLOOD PRESSURE, DIABETES, HEART DISEASE). IS IT SAFE FOR ME TO EXERCISE?
Exercise is safe for almost everyone. In fact, studies show that people with arthritis, high blood pressure, diabetes, or heart disease benefit from regular exercise and physical activity. In some cases, exercise can improve some of these conditions. You will want to talk with your doctor about how your health condition might affect your ability to be active.

IF I'M OVERWEIGHT OR OBESE, WHAT KINDS OF PHYSICAL ACTIVITY CAN I DO?
You can do all kinds of physical activities. Try walking, water exercises, or weight lifting. Anything that gets you moving — even for only a few minutes a day in the beginning — is a healthy start. Very large people may face unique challenges. For example, you may not

be able to bend or move easily, or you may feel self-conscious. Facing these challenges is hard — but it can be done. Feel good about what you can do, and pat yourself on the back for trying. It should get easier.[6]

IS IT TRUE THAT IT DOESN'T MATTER HOW MUCH YOU WEIGH AS LONG AS YOU ARE FIT?

According to Shape Up America, research has shown that a group of overweight men who were fit were more likely to outlive thin men who were out of shape. So being thin is no substitute for being fit. Fat is a threat if it is located in your belly. If you also have other risk factors for disease such as high blood pressure, high cholesterol, or high blood sugar, then it's time to lose a few pounds in addition to getting fit.

IF I LIFT WEIGHTS, WILL MY MUSCLES GET BIGGER?

Whether or not a person is able to build bigger muscles depends on three primary factors: genetics, gender, and training intensity. Genetics are manifested in muscle fiber type (hypertrophy); people with predominantly fast-twitch fibers acquire larger muscles more easily than people with slow-twitch fibers. Concerning gender, males acquire larger muscles than females do, because males have greater amounts of testosterone and other hormones that influence protein metabolism. Training intensity is the only factor you can control. Hypertrophy results from an increase in the number of contractile proteins (actin and myosin, produced by the body in response to training), which in turn enhance the size of the muscle fibers. If the training goal is hypertrophy, the load lifted should be at least 80 percent of the one-repetition, as a general rule. If you are not interested in developing larger muscles, keep the load less than 80 percent. However, hypertrophy can be stimulated any time the training intensity is high enough to overload the muscle. Thus, in someone who has never lifted weights before, 60 percent of 1

RM may be enough to cause slight hypertrophy, especially if he/she is predisposed to hypertrophy by having a large proportion of fast-twitch fibers.[16]

HOW DO I GET A FLAT STOMACH OR "SIX-PACK?"

Genetics also play a significant role in whether a flat stomach or "six-pack" can be obtained; strength training and cardiovascular exercise can help. According to Jason Karp, PhD., the abdominals are just like any other muscle group: for their definition to become visible, they must grow larger, and the fat that lies over them must decrease. What makes the definition of the abdominals so difficult to see is that they are situated in the area of the body that contains the most fat. So, in order to get a "six pack", you must lose the bulk of the fat in your stomach first. Karp says that most people do not do nearly enough cardiovascular exercise to decrease their body fat percentage to a point where they would see their abdominals. The role of diet must be considered in this effort since those with a flat stomach or six-pack have a very low percentage of body fat. Karp also notes that abdominal crunches are just as effective as any piece of equipment to train the abdominal muscles. As you improve their abdominal strength, you can make crunches more demanding by performing them on a movable surface, such as a resistance ball.

DO I NEED TO TAKE DIETARY SUPPLEMENTS?

Supplements for losing fat or building muscle are rapidly becoming popular. Jason Karp, PhD., says that although claims that "fat-burning" supplements will decrease body fat by increasing either mobilization or oxidation of free fatty acids (FFAs), they are faulty. Exercise alone increases the muscles' capacity to oxidize FFAs. For those who eat a balanced diet, there is no evidence that muscle-building supplements, including protein powders and amino acids, build muscle mass (Clarkson 1998; Eichner et al. 1999). The few supplements whose muscle-building potential is supported by research (e.g., creatine) are effective mostly in elite athletes who have undergone many years of training (Eichner et al. 1999).

HOW DO I GET RID OF MY FLABBY ARMS?

One of the biggest exercise myths is that you can lose fat in an area of the body by strength training or exercising that specific body part. Jason Karp, PhD., says the truth is that "spot reducing" and "spot toning" do not work, because you cannot dictate from where your body will decide to oxidize fat, nor can you change fat into muscle.

Doing tricep press-downs will not decrease the amount of fat you have on the backs of your arms any more than doing crunches will decrease the amount of fat you have on your stomach.

As you age, your skin will become less elastic and thus conform less to the arms. So "flabby arms" are somewhat a product of age. Any exercise that decreases body fat percentage will help you lose fat on your arms, just as it will help you lose fat from other areas of the body.[16]

STATISTICS & FACTS

According to the Centers for Disease Control and Prevention, some Americans are getting enough exercise, but too many are not.

- About 1 in 5 (21%) adults meet the 2008 Physical Activity Guidelines.

- Less than 3 in 10 high school students gets at least 60 minutes of physical activity every day.

- Physical activity can improve health. People who are physically active tend to live longer and have a lower risk of heart disease, stroke, type 2 diabetes, depression, and some cancers. Physical activity can also help with weight control and may improve academic achievement in students.

- Inactive adults have a higher risk of early death, heart disease, stroke, type 2 diabetes, depression, and some cancers.

Rates of activity and inactivity vary across states and regions

- Americans living in the South are less likely to be physically active than Americans living in the West, Northeast and Midwest regions of the country.

Some groups are more physically active than others

- Men (54%) are more likely than women (46%) to meet the 2008 Physical Activity Guideline for aerobic activity.

- Younger adults are more likely to meet the 2008 Physical Activity Guideline for aerobic activity than older adults.

PART THREE
WEIGHT LOSS

For the Love of Living

Chapter Eleven
INTRODUCTION TO WEIGHT LOSS

Simple, basic nutrition is the starting point for losing weight. It is not only the recipe for health and longevity – it has been shown as the best way to lose weight in a manner that will enable you to keep it off.

After learning the basics of nutrition and healthy eating from our nutrition guide, take the next step towards your weight loss goals with this plan. We use the same principles talked about in the nutrition guide, but adapt them to weight loss and include a custom workout regimen to accompany it.

You'll learn things such as how our bodies lose weight, and the core science behind it that marketing companies won't tell you. Find out how to lose your excess pounds and keep them off with a plan that does not require any magic pill, powder, or program. We provide a gradual process for weight loss that doesn't use extreme limiting of certain foods, and which you can adjust to your liking.

This is a weight loss plan for everyone. It is designed to be adjustable to your needs and suitable for a long-term approach to weight management.

Start today on a delicious journey to eating that you will enjoy and that can last you a lifetime!

THE SCIENCE OF WEIGHT LOSS

So many people are trying to sell the secret to weight loss – it's no wonder that there is so much confusion on the subject. Health and weight control are one of people's greatest concerns today, so it is easy to target that market. Is it possible that the key to losing weight can be free? That it doesn't require a special formula or program? It's true.

It is important to note that every individual's journey to health and weight control is unique, and it is sometimes necessary to try various approaches to see what works for you. However, you can follow these basic principles to understand the science of weight loss.

To lose weight, you must consume fewer calories than you expend.

You burn calories every day just going about your normal activities, including the internal functions of your body. The food that you eat provides the necessary energy (calories) to fuel this activity. If you consume fewer calories than the amount expended, you lose weight; if you consume more than expended, you gain weight. If your body is not functioning correctly, (because of a thyroid or adrenal problem, for instance), you may be gaining or losing weight because of that condition. See your doctor for any such problem.

Not all calories are equal

Did you know that your body only stores fat when insulin is released into your bloodstream? Insulin is released when we eat empty calories like sugar and refined flours. In light of this, we can recognize that neither sugar nor fat is entirely bad for you, but if you're pairing them together often (i.e. donuts, deep fried foods & pizza) it can be detrimental to your health.

On the other hand, some foods facilitate weight loss. According to Harvard Health, a diet based on plant foods and healthy fats has been proven by extensive research to have the best influence on preventing chronic illness and high blood pressure. These foods also keep you feeling full longer and more satisfied with fewer calories.

We have to ask ourselves the question of whether or not the calories we consume are beneficial to our long-term health and bodies. If we are only consuming "empty calories" such as white flour, sugars, deep-fried items, and high-fat foods such as cured meats, we are not only making it hard to manage weight but are also missing all the benefits of whole foods. Plant sources and healthy fats offer a myriad of the vitamins, minerals, fiber, and phytochemicals that our bodies need to function and fight off disease.

Basics of a diet conducive to long-term health & weight control:
- Plant foods as the primary source of daily calories. These include fruits, vegetables, whole grains, nuts, and legumes (like beans, peas, and lentils), with a preference for foods that are fresh and minimally processed to preserve nutrients. Olive oil as the principal source of fat calories. Some research suggests that extra-virgin olive oil may contain beneficial substances that other oils lose in processing.

- Low to moderate amounts of cheese and yogurt with meals.

- Minimal amounts of red meat, with moderate amounts of fish and poultry as the preferred sources of animal protein.

- Small amounts of sweets, eaten occasionally; fresh fruit with meals, instead of desserts.

- For those who drink alcohol, wine consumed in low to moderate amounts, usually with meals.

Diet plus exercise makes it easier to keep the weight off longer.

You've heard that you should combine exercise with your diet plan in order to see results. But did you know that is not the only reason why you should exercise with your diet? According to Harvard Health, the body reacts to weight loss as if it were starving and, in response, slows its metabolism. When your metabolism slows, you burn fewer calories – even at rest. When you burn fewer calories, three things can happen. If you continue eating fewer calories, your weight loss may slow, or you might stop losing weight altogether. If you then increase your calorie consumption, you may actually gain weight more quickly than you have in the past. The solution is to increase your physical activity; doing so will counteract the metabolic slow-down caused by reducing calories.

A regular habit of exercise not only helps you burn calories but also increases the rate at which you burn calories at rest! According to Harvard Health, scientists are finding that the bodies of people who stay active throughout their lives improve all the way down to the insides of their cells. For example, active people's mitochondria—the energy-producing power plants within each cell—become highly efficient at burning fatty fuel, even when that person is at rest. This doesn't mean you have to run marathons—just 30 minutes of moderate activity nearly every day will do the trick.

There is a realistic amount of weight that you can expect to lose in a given time, and then keep it off.

It takes approximately 3,500 calories to equal a pound. Cut about 500 calories a day for a week, and you should lose 1 lb. It is not recommended to cut more than 1,000 calories a day. Therefore, the safe amount of weight that you can expect to lose in a week is 1-2 pounds. The downside to cutting more calories is that it will lead to significant deprivation, which will soon leave you feeling hungry and wanting to quit or cheat. Secondly, the vast contrast between such a strict diet and a regular high-calorie diet usually causes dieters to regain their original weight, or even more, when they return to their normal style of eating.

If you have excess weight, you may lose your first 5 or so pounds quickly. However, dieticians recommend that if you are trying to lose more than a few pounds, you should see weight loss as a gradual process in order to then keep it off. Many weight loss successes happen over a period of several months.

Diets that promise significant weight loss in an unrealistic time frame are often not concerned with long-term weight loss, but are simply a part of the $33 billion dieting industry.2

Sudden changes in diet can slow your metabolism, cause neurological stress (making restricted foods much more appealing), and cause hormone changes that will affect how full you feel. This is why it is recommended to ease your way into a diet. Use our plan to choose a phase from which to begin – first by reducing portion size, then eating more whole foods, and then choosing leaner foods. You will see much more success by viewing weight loss as a long-term goal.

It is also important to recognize that merely restricting calories is not the only key to success for weight loss. Age, gender, weight, activity level, and other factors also come into play. Many people plateau after several months of dieting and need to reorganize their efforts, such as adding more exercise or changing up their routine.

Making a lifestyle of healthy choices and exercise is the best way to maintain your weight (and it doesn't have to be extreme).

Losing weight is a difficult journey, and once you've done the hard work of losing it, you want to keep it off. The best way to do this is to make healthy eating and being active a lifestyle choice. This may sound difficult at first but can be handled with balance. We recommend using the 80/20 rule. Aim to eat healthily 80% of the time and eat outside of that habit 20% of the time. Depriving yourself of treats and the foods you love is hard to maintain and usually leads to bingeing.

The key is to understand what healthy choices look like, and learn how to fit them into your life. The recommended diet plan in this guide is a more lean, focused version of the lifestyle plan, which is why the transition off of that plan works so well.

According to The Psychology of Eating, most of us can change our eating habits for a week or two, sometimes even for a month, but most often dietary-induced changes are merely external ones. "Eat this, and don't eat that." What we eat is important, but just changing the type of food we ingest does not necessarily create long lasting change. It doesn't touch the deep-rooted beliefs, patterns, and behaviors that inform our food choices and eating habits in the first place.

If a diet only focuses on food choices and doesn't touch upon the "why" of those choices, you will keep reaching for foods that diminish your energy and health and will be stuck working only on the surface level. In order to make sustainable changes in your eating habits, you need to explore why and how you eat, and who you in relation to your eating.

80/20 RULE

Eat nutritiously 80% of the time.

Allow yourself to eat your favorite

less-nutritious foods 20% of the time.

For the Love of Living

Chapter Twelve
SET A GOAL

Where your mind is set, your body will follow. Take some time to answer these questions and set some goals that will keep you motivated along the way:

NO-LIMIT GOALS
- If your life could be anything you imagined, what would it be like? Would you have more energy, be more involved in your family's lives, climb mountains, feel better about yourself?
- What would you be doing?
- How would you feel?
- What would your priorities be?

LONG-TERM GOALS
- Where would you like to be in 5-10 years?
- What would you wish to look and feel like?
- What would your lifestyle be?

SHORT-TERM GOALS
- What steps do you need to take to reach these long-term goals?
- What do you need to start doing?
- What is within your control to do?
- What phase will you start at in this plan?

WEIGHT LOSS & FITNESS GOALS
Remember to consider that the healthy weight to lose is 1-2 pounds a week, and sometimes you will lose less or go through plateaus. When gaining muscle, the number on the scale is not as revealing as inches.

- What is your dream weight?
- What is your **long-term** weight goal (include date to accomplish)?
- What is your **short-term** weight goal (include date to accomplish)?

For the Love of Living

Chapter Thirteen
THE PLAN

CHOOSE YOUR PHASE

PHASE 1
Eat Less + Exercise More
Don't put too much pressure on yourself to dive into dieting. Simply start eating less to make later adjustments easier, and move more - walk instead of ride, add an after dinner walk, or spend an hour playing with your kids.

PHASE 2
Focus on eating whole foods + Get 2-1/2 hours of moderate-vigorous intensity exercise weekly (Example 1 or 2 workout).
Ease into the challenge with this step-by-step approach:

- **Week 1:** Eliminate high-fat dairy, refined sugar, and highly processed foods. (Choose a few meals from the recipe lists and plan to make them this week). Do the example 1 workout.

- **Week 2:** Build on the successes of the previous week! Eliminate high- fat meats. Do the Example 1 meal plan and workout.

- **Week 3:** Keep up the good work! Do the Example 2 meal plan and workout.

- **Week 4:** Congratulations! You have advanced to the final Phase! (Repeat the Example 1 meal plan or create your own with the sample recipes for as many weeks as you would like to keep losing weight). Do the Example 2 workout.

PHASE 3
Do the Last Pounds Meal Plan or eliminate added sugar, high fat meats, refined carbs and dairy + Get 2-1/2 hours of moderate-vigorous intensity exercise with strength training weekly (Example 3 workout).

TIPS

PANTRY MAKEOVER
Set yourself up for success by eliminating unhealthy foods from your home and replace them with healthy choices. If the bad choices are not there, you are less likely to be tempted by them and will be more inclined to grab a healthy snack. Fill your pantry with staples from the healthy pantry grocery list in the index, and snacks from the snack list. (Apart of Nutrition Guide – direct accordingly).

SNACK SMART
To help curb hunger, we recommend having a nutritious snack

between meals. You can ruin your dieting efforts by grabbing a cookie or can of soda. Instead, choose a piece of fruit or some nuts and cheese. See the snack list for delicious suggestions! If you find that you are not hungry between meals anymore, you can eliminate the snack.

A GUIDE TO CHEATING

When you're dieting, it's ok to cheat every now and then. If you deprive yourself of too much, you will sabotage your efforts and end up throwing your diet out the door. The important thing is knowing how to cheat without ruining your diet. A great way to do this is to include your cheat into your calorie count for the day. If you know that you will be going out for dinner and want to make room for dessert, plan ahead and eat much leaner during the day. Sometimes you will go over your calories, and that is ok! We would recommend that you only allow this to happen one day a week or every other week. If you cheat all weekend, you'll spend the whole next week making up for it and will struggle to see results.

FIND FOODS & RECIPES YOU ENJOY

Everyone has different tastes and to some people, salads and avocado may sound terrible! Even if you don't like salad or enjoy raw vegetables, there are ways to eat nutritiously – you just have to find what you like. Take the time to decide what foods you like and how you like them prepared. This will be key to your success. If you don't care for salad greens, place your vegetables atop a bed of cooked rice. If you don't care for raw vegetables, make a stir-fry or pop your veggies in the broiler with a little olive oil and salt. As you try new foods, you will enjoy expanding your culinary horizons.

CHANGE UP YOUR ROUTINE REGULARLY
Since weight loss should be considered a long-term goal, it is important to keep variety in your plan so that you don't get sick of what you're eating and doing. Find new recipes that you like and different ways and places to exercise. This will keep you motivated as well as contribute to making it a lifestyle change that you can maintain.

SET GOALS FOR YOURSELF & TRACK YOUR EFFORTS
You've heard it before; you can't accomplish what you don't determine. Take some time to fill out the goal-setting section of this guide before getting started with your weight loss endeavor. Taking that step is vital to your success. By setting a goal, you make a commitment to yourself as well as a concrete accomplishment to work towards – whether that be feeling better, losing 10 pounds, or being able to play with your grandkids. Likewise, tracking your efforts will help you to keep your eye on your goal, and you can re-evaluate as needed.

GET SUPPORT
In any important endeavor, it is vital to have support. You may decide to include a friend who wants to get healthier as well, or simply share your goal in order to be held accountable. You will have much more success by sharing it than by keeping it to yourself. Choose a person (or a few) that you will ask to support you in your journey.

MEAL PLAN GUIDELINES

You can use these guidelines to create your diet and meal plans with the recipes in the index, or create your own plan.

- The meals in this plan contain a balance of protein, carbohydrates, and healthy fat.

- PROTEIN servings are approximately the size of your fist (1/2 cup cooked)

- CARBOHYDRATE servings are approximately the size of your fist (1 slice of whole grain bread, ½ whole grains cooked, 1 piece of fruit).
   When cooking grains, ¼ cup dry = ½ cup cooked

- FAT servings are approximately 1 tbsp. of a healthy fat (olive, canola, avocado, nut, safflower, or sunflower oils) or about 8 walnuts per serving.

- Vegetables are unlimited

- Fruit should be considered a carbohydrate when dieting

- Water: The daily recommendation is 13 - 8oz. servings for men, 9 - 8oz. servings for women (Amount needed depends on a number of factors including your size, activity level, and the weather).

STILL HUNGRY?
- If you find that you are still hungry because you're adjusting to smaller quantities, increase your vegetables and protein. Your vegetable allowance is unlimited so eat up! If that doesn't satisfy, add some healthy fats (1 serving to start). Do not add carbohydrates, which will leave you feeling hungrier and will not contribute to weight loss.

- If you find that you are still hungry because you are working really hard or exercising more, than you can try drinking a scoop of whey protein mixed with water, and a piece of fruit like an apple or banana. Eat as many vegetables as you like; if you are still hungry, you can increase your protein servings by 2 ounces at meals. Reach for protein-rich foods such as nuts for your snack between meals.

SEE RECIPES AT THE END OF PART I - NUTRITION

MEAL PLAN - *Example 1*

SUNDAY
B – Oatmeal w/ cottage cheese and blueberries
L – Curried Tuna Salad Sandwich w/ avocado and whole grain toast
D – Lemon-Basil Butter Chicken w/Brussels sprouts & rice

MONDAY
B – Scrambled eggs, avocado and toast
L – Chicken, Brussels sprouts and Quinoa Salad
D – Sesame-Roasted Turnips and Barley

TUESDAY
B – Apple-Berry Smoothie
L – Chopped Avocado, Feta and Barley Salad
D – Soy Salmon with Stir-Fried Quinoa

WEDNESDAY
B – Vegetable omelet
L – Cucumber Salmon Salad
D – Spinach and Feta Pie with Chickpea Flour Crust, side salad

THURSDAY
B – Toast with almond butter and bananas
L – Spinach amd Feta Pie with Chickpea Flour Crust, side salad
D – Vegetable Bean Fajitas

FRIDAY
B – Oatmeal with Greek yogurt and berries
L – Garden salad with black beans
D – Tomato and White Bean Soup, side salad with quinoa

SATURDAY
B – Vegetable and potato omelet
L – Tomato and White Bean Soup with side salad
D – Simple Chicken Curry with side salad

Example 1: Leaner, yet still flavorful choices using leftovers from supper for the following day's lunch.

Water: Aim to drink 13 - 8oz. servings for men daily, 9 - 8oz. servings for women daily

SEE RECIPES AT THE END OF PART I - NUTRITION

MEAL PLAN - *Example 2*

SUNDAY
B - One cup non-fat plain Greek yogurt, 3/4 cup blueberries, 2 tbsp. pecans
L - Chicken Harvest Soup
D - Easy Vegetarian Chili

MONDAY
B - Hot whole grain cereal with blueberries
L - Easy Vegetarian Chili with side salad
D - Blackened Fish Tacos with Avocado-Cilantro Sauce

TUESDAY
B - 2 scrambled eggs w/ bell pepper, 2 slices whole-grain toast, 1 orange
L - Blackened Fish Tacos with Avocado-Cilantro Sauce
D - Quick Chicken Gumbo

WEDNESDAY
B - Oatmeal cooked with apples and bananas
L - Quick Chicken Gumbo with side salad
D - Spice-Rubbed Chicken over Sauteed Spinach and Whole Grains

THURSDAY
B - Whole-grain toast with nut butter and ½ cup skim milk
L - BBQ Chicken Salad
D - Mushroom and Wild Rice Black Bean Burger with side salad

FRIDAY
B - 1 egg over-easy on toast with avocado
L - Turkey breast on whole-grain toast w/ lettuce and tomato, 1 tbsp. light mayo
D - 3 oz. pork tenderloin, 1 medium baked sweet potato, ½ cup stir-fried broccoli, cauliflower, & carrots, 1 cup skim milk

SATURDAY
B - Whole-grain bagel or toast with ricotta & strawberry preserves, yogurt & fruit
L - Lg. mixed greens salad, 1 small pita w/1 cup stir-fried vegetables, cucumber and tomato slices, 3 oz. salmon; drizzle w/ 2 tbsp olive oil and 1 tbsp red wine vinegar.
D - Turkey Meatloaf with baked sweet potato and garden salad

Example 2: May choose one snack from the snack list in between meals. Side salad: Greens, with any desired vegetables, 1 tbsp. oil, 1 tbsp. vinegar, pinch salt & pepper

Water: Aim to drink 13 - 8oz. servings for men daily, 9 - 8oz. servings for women daily.

The Plan

SEE RECIPES AT THE END OF PART I - NUTRITION

MEAL PLAN - *Last Pounds*

SUNDAY
B - 2 eggs scrambled with 1 tbsp. olive oil
L - Tuna Salad on whole-grain toast
D - Chicken Stir-Fry, baked asparagus

MONDAY
B - 2 eggs scrambled with 1 tbsp. olive oil
L - BBQ Chicken Salad
D - Salmon Steak Florentine

TUESDAY
B - 2 eggs scrambled with 1 tbsp. olive oil
L - Broiled Shrimp w/ Lemon, side salad
D - Chicken Burger, baked sweet potato, side salad drizzled w/ 1 tbsp oil, 1 tbsp vinegar, pinch of salt and pepper

WEDNESDAY
B - 2 eggs scrambled with 1 tbsp. olive oil
L - Turkey, 1/2 baked sweet potato, side salad drizzled w/ 1 tbsp oil, 1 tbsp vinegar, pinch of salt and pepper
D - Grilled fish & broccoli

THURSDAY
B - 2 eggs scrambled with 1 tbsp. olive oil
L - Grilled fish and steamed spinach
D - Mexican Stuffed Chicken

FRIDAY
B - 2 eggs scrambled with 1 tbsp. olive oil
L - BBQ Tuna
D - Turkey Kabobs and Easy Vegetarian Chili

SATURDAY
B - 2 eggs scrambled with 1 tbsp. olive oil
L - Chicken Stew
D - Stir-Fried Fish Filets

Breakfast: Wait 5 hours after breakfast for lunch
Lunch: Wait 6 hours after lunch to eat dinner
No Snacks in between meals with this plan
Unlimited amount of vegetable soup or caffeine-free tea
Water: Aim to drink 13 - 8oz. servings for men daily, 9 - 8oz. servings for women daily

SUBSTITUTES

Use any of these substitutes in the meal plans to cater to your taste.

SAMPLE PROTEIN
- 6 oz. fish
- 6 oz. poultry (chicken, turkey)
- 2 whole eggs
- 5 egg whites
- 4 oz. red meat (counts as your fat serving as well)
- ½ cup Greek yogurt
- ½ cup hummus (may count as fat serving as well – check label)

SAMPLE CARBOHYDRATES
- Vegetable (other than potato which is considered a starchy carb), unlimited
- Small orange
- Small apple
- Oatmeal (1/2 cup cooked)
- Quinoa, brown rice or other whole grain (1/2 cup cooked)
- 1 piece whole grain bread
- ½ cup beans
- Small sweet potato

SAMPLE FATS
- 1 tbsp. healthy fat (olive, canola, avocado, nut, safflower or sunflower oils)
- Raw nuts – approximately 8 if replacing a fat
- 1 tbsp. almond, cashew or other nut butters
- 1 tbsp. avocado

SNACK OPTIONS

Choose: Whole foods like fruit, vegetables, nuts, seeds and low-fat dairy.

* Note that fruit juice is not on this list. There is a very concentrated amount of sugar (even if natural) in juice, more than if you eat the recommended amount of fresh fruit. If you prefer juice, squeeze a ½ cup of fresh fruit yourself.

- Handful of grapes with a slice of hard cheese (cheddar, Swiss)
- Half an avocado with salt
- ½ grapefruit
- ¼ cup unsalted nuts or seeds
- Carrot and celery sticks
- 2 tbsp. hummus with 1 cup fresh vegetables
- 1 oz. Swiss cheese
- 1½ oz. trail mix with dried fruit, dark chocolate and walnuts
- 1 banana, sliced and spread with 1 tbsp. nut butter
- ½ orange
- ½ cup Greek yogurt and ½ cup berries
- 1 apple
- 1 cup of popcorn with dusting of dark chocolate shavings
- A smoothie (1 cup fruit, water & ice)
- 1½ oz. dark chocolate
- ½ cup of low-fat cottage cheese or ricotta and vegetables for dipping
- 1½ oz. cocoa dusted almonds and dried cherries

EXERCISE PLANS

Exercise is key to losing weight and maintaining it! See *Chapter 11* for more information about why exercise keeps you from reaching weight-loss plateaus.

These workout plans are designed for our weight-loss program. You can use them, or substitute other activities that you prefer.

Keep in mind that levels of exertion will vary for every person. For those just starting out, a brisk 15 minute walk may be a moderate level activity. See *Chapter 6* for suggestions of activities for your level.

CIRCUITS
By Corrie Trotter – Certified Personal Trainer, American College of Sports Medicine

A circuit is a simple way to get both strength training and cardiovascular work done in one workout. With little to no breaks between exercises, your heart rate should stay elevated in the same way it does when doing a cardiovascular exercise like walking fast or running. Circuits can be made from a combination of nearly any exercises, but the most efficient way to build a simple circuit is to use exercises that work primary muscle groups or multiple muscle groups at the same time.

Circuits can be done by time or repetitions. They should always be done after a short warm up of 5 – 10 minutes.

The following sequence is an example of a circuit one could do at home. After each exercise, try to go directly to the next exercise, only breaking when noted.

The Plan

CIRCUIT BY REPETITIONS: 10 - 12 REPETITIONS OF EACH EXERCISE

CIRCUIT WORKOUT ONE

EXERCISE	NUMBER OF REPS
Body Weight Squat	10 -12
Plank or Modified Plant	30 sec. or 2 sets of 15 sec.
Heel Raises	10 - 12
Push-up or Modified Push-up	10 - 12
Walking lunges	10 - 12 each leg
Reverse Crunches	30 sec. per side
Side Lunges	10 - 12 per leg
Jumping Jacks	20 - 30

REST 1 MINUTE

REPEAT FULL WORKOUT 2 - 3 TIMES

EXERCISE EXPLANATIONS

Body Weight Squat - with feet shoulder width apart, lower into a chair position keeping your chest up and body weight pressing into your heels. Return to standing. Repeat.

Plank – Lying chest to the ground, bend your elbows and rest your weight on your forearms, not your hands. Lift your hips off the ground and tighten your abdomen by trying to pull your belly button toward your spine.

Modified Plank – Laying chest to the ground, place your hand on the ground under your shoulders and extend your arms pushing your chest off the ground with arms fully extended. Keep knees bent and in contact with the ground. Abdomen should be engaged and body should still form a straight line from the head to the knee (try not to bend at the hip crease).

Heel Raises – Stand with feet shoulder width apart. Raise your heels off the ground and try to pause while extended. Lower back to the ground. Repeat.

Push-up or Modified Push-up - From kneeling, place hands on the ground in front of you and shift your weight forward, extending your legs fully into a plank. With your hands 45 inches wider than your shoulders, lower your body to the ground then press back up into plank by extending your elbows. Repeat.

Modified Push-up - from kneeling, place your hands on the ground in front of you, slightly wider than your shoulders. Shift your weight forward and allow your hips to straighten so that there is no bend at the hip crease. Lower your upper body to just above the ground then press back up extending the elbows until arms are straight. Repeat.

Walking Lunges - step out with one foot and lunge with body weight moving downwards. Press back up by pushing off the back leg to meet the front. Repeat on opposite side.

Reverse Crunches – Lying on your back, place your hands flat underneath the lowest part of the back for support. Pull the knees into the chest, then extend back to the floor. Repeat.

Side Lunges – Standing with hips shoulder-width apart and knees slightly bent, step out wide (laterally) with one foot, keeping toes pointed forward. Lower body by bending at the knee, keeping weight in the heel. Push off bent leg to return to standing. Repeat on opposite side.

The Plan

CIRCUIT BY REPETITIONS: 10 - 12 REPETITIONS OF EACH EXERCISE

CIRCUIT WORKOUT TWO

EXERCISE	NUMBER OF REPS
Weighted Squat	10 - 12
Overhead Press	10 - 12
Seated Russian Twist	10 - 12
Rest 30 seconds - 1 minute	
Walking Lunges	10 - 12 each leg
Flat Back, bent over row	10 - 12
Full Extension Crunch	10 - 12
Rest 30 seconds - 1 minute	
Sumo Squat w/ Pulse	10 - 12
Push-up	10 - 12
Straight Leg Raises	10 - 12
Rest 30 seconds - 1 minute	
Speed Skater Lunge	10 - 12 each leg
Overhead Triceps Extension	10 - 12
Lying Hip Raises	10 - 12
Jump Rope / Jumping Jacks	50

REST 1 MINUTE

REPEAT FULL WORKOUT 3 TIMES

EXERCISE EXPLANATIONS

Weighted Squat - Hold weights up at chest level with feet shoulder width apart, lower into a chair position keeping your chest up and body weight pressing into your heels. Return to standing. Repeat.

Overhead Press – While standing, hold the weights up and out at each side making an "L" or right angle, press them to meet each other overhead and return to right angle. Repeat.

Seated Russian Twist – while seated, hold one dumbbell at your chest. With bent legs, lean backward until tension is felt in the abdomen. From this point rotate entire upper body to the left, then back to center, then to the right while keeping the hips and legs as still as possible.

Walking Lunges – Carrying a weight in each hand, step out with one foot and lunge with body weight moving downwards. Press back up by pushing off the back leg to meet the front. Repeat on opposite side.

Flat Back, Bent Over Row – Holding a weight in each hand, bend from the waist keeping the back straight, with a slight bend in the knees. Place the weights on the outside of the knees palms up. Pull the arms to the outside of the body near the rib-cage using a rowing motion then release back down while maintaining a flat back.

Full Extension Crunch – While lying on your back, fully extend your legs and arms holding each slightly above the ground. Simultaneously pull your knees to your chest and arms to your knees, then fully extend. Repeat.

Sumo Squat w/ Pulse – Hold weights at chest level and feet wider than shoulder width apart, toes pointing slightly outward. Lower into a squat position keeping the chest up, pulse slightly while lowered then return to standing pressing hips slightly forward and squeezing the glute muscles. Repeat.

Push-up – From kneeling, place hands on the ground in front of you and shift your weight forward, extending your legs fully into a plank. With your hands 4-5 inches wider than your shoulders, lower your body to the ground then press back up into plank by extending your elbows. Repeat. To do a modified push-up, from kneeling place your hands on the ground in front of your, slightly wider than your shoulders. Shift your weight forward and allow your hips to straighten so that there is no bend at the hip crease. Lower your upper body to just above the ground then press back up extending the elbows until arms are straight. Repeat.

Straight Leg Raises – While lying on the ground, place hands under the lower back for support. Lift legs into the air so that the sole of the foot is facing the ceiling. Lower both legs slowly 4-6 inches above ground then lift again. Repeat.

Speed Skater Lunge – From standing, lift right leg and place on the ground at an angle behind the left leg, lowering into a lunge. Press off the right foot, bringing it back to standing. Repeat on the opposite side. (Optional – hold weights at chest level for added resistance).

Overhead Triceps Extension – While standing, lift one weight with both hands straight above your head. Bending at the elbow, lower the weight behind the back to shoulder level then extend the arms bringing the weight back up overhead. Repeat.

Lying Hip Raises – While lying on your back, bend at the knees, placing your feet flat on the ground and hip width apart. Using the glute muscles, hamstrings and lower back muscles lift the hips off the ground toward the ceiling. Gently lower back to the ground and repeat.

To do the same circuit by time, simply do each exercise for 30 seconds, and then rest for 10 seconds. After completing three exercises, take a full 30 seconds to 1-minute break.

To increase difficulty, try increasing from 10 – 12 reps. Once you reach 12 reps each, you can increase the weight by 2 – 5 lbs. for upper body exercises, 5 – 10 lbs. for lower body exercises. You can also increase difficulty by shortening the rest periods.

FINAL THOUGHTS

You don't have to count your calories to have success in weight loss; however, logging your general progress can be key to keeping you on track. This works in a couple of different ways - by documenting your progress, you can see what works for you and what doesn't. Comparing different exercises and the foods that you are eating each week will remind you of your goal and inspire you to keep going. Have fun and enjoy the journey to your new healthy lifestyle!

FREQUENTLY ASKED
QUESTIONS

HOW LONG DOES IT TAKE TO SEE RESULTS IF YOU EAT HEALTHY?[2]

Immediate

When you begin eating healthy, you'll feel certain changes immediately. You will feel less heavy and bloated after a meal when you give up high-calorie, fat-laden foods, and you may experience fewer incidences of indigestion when you eat smaller portions. Choosing whole grains over refined carbs will help keep your blood sugar steady throughout the day, so you may experience less of a mid-afternoon slump. Because you'll be feeding your body usable nutrients instead of empty calories, you may notice an increase in energy and alertness.

Next

Within a few days to a few weeks, you may notice a decrease in water retention and bloating as the high water and fiber content of a healthy diet kicks in. You may have a small drop in weight, and your energy levels will increase as your vitamin supply becomes fully stocked. Choosing and preparing the right foods will become easier, and you may find yourself enjoying and even craving healthy foods. Your junk food cravings may fade. Your new, lighter feeling and increased energy levels may increase your desire to move, and you'll find yourself looking forward to a daily workout.

Soon

After a few months, your weight may be noticeably lower, and extra pounds continue to drop at a slow but steady rate. High blood pressure may decrease, and cholesterol levels drop. Your skin will look better from the constant influx of vitamins, minerals, and water, and you may notice a decrease in appetite. Food can go from being a focal point in your life to just a way to fuel your body. You may notice less joint pain as your reduced weight requires less effort to move. Healthy eating goes from being a diet to being a way of life.

Eventually

If you keep at it, you'll notice what a pleasure it is to use your muscles. Lean protein feeds your muscle fibers without weighing you down with excess fat, so simple tasks like carrying groceries won't be as difficult. Your new lower weight remains steady because you are only giving your body what it needs and no more. Your higher energy levels and nourished body make exercise a stress-reducing escape rather than a chore, and improved alertness and mental clarity allow you to be more productive because you can finally focus on the task at hand. Your risk of chronic disease is lowered, and you may begin to look, move, and feel younger than you are.

*By Ilyse Schapiro, MS, RD, CDN, co-author of Should I Scoop My Bagel & The Editors of Eat This, Not That! * Eatthis.com*

WHY CAN'T I STOP EATING THE BREAD FROM THE BREADBASKET?

This magnetic force isn't really your fault. Since the breadbasket at most restaurants tends to be filled with white bread, there's hardly any fiber in it. They're basically putting an enormous amount of sugar in front of you, which is why it's so addictive. How many times have you said, "I'll just have five jelly beans," which turns into fifty and suddenly you can't stop eating them? It's the same with the breadbasket. Either tell them not to put the breadbasket down on the table, or just take one piece and have them take the rest away. Alternatively, order an appetizer. House salads, vegetable soup, and shrimp cocktail are great options.

I HAVE SALADS FOR LUNCH EVERY DAY, AND I'M STILL NOT LOSING WEIGHT. WHAT AM I DOING WRONG?

First of all, you should not have the same thing for lunch every day. You change your exercise routine to challenge different muscles and keep yourself from getting bored; you should do the same with your meals. In fact, doing so helps keep your metabolism in high gear.

Just because a meal has the word salad in it doesn't automatically make it a healthy or low-calorie choice. To find out how your salad ranks, start by taking an inventory of what you've put in your bowl: what kinds of toppings, how much dressing, and how big is it? A good rule to follow when eating a salad is to stay away from iceberg lettuce, which has very few (if any) nutrients and fiber. Instead, use more nutritious greens, like kale, spinach, romaine, arugula, or mesclun. Fill your salad with unlimited veggies, but avoid peas and corn, as those tend to be starchy. Watch the extras such as cheese, nuts, seeds, crunchy things (like wontons, noodles, croutons, bacon bits) and dried fruits (raisins, craisins). Choose a lean protein such as grilled chicken, shrimp, turkey, tofu, eggs, or salmon, and avoid fried, breaded, and processed meats. Get a full-fat dressing (you need fat to absorb the most nutrients) on the side and stick to two tablespoons or less.

WHAT SHOULD I DO WHEN I'M STILL HUNGRY AFTER DINNER AND ALL I WANT TO DO IS RAID THE FRIDGE?

This is one of those times that you need to have a serious talk with yourself. Say to yourself: "Am I really hungry or am I just thinking of food because it's a bad habit I've gotten myself into over the years?"

If you end up evading your own question, try drinking a glass of water. Many times, dehydration mimics hunger, so you may actually be mistaking your want for food with your need for liquids. After you have a drink, try waiting a few minutes and distract yourself, then see if you're still hungry. If the urge passes, then you've just saved yourself calories, and you probably were not hungry to begin with. If you're still famished, try to figure out why. Before the meal, did you drink too much (juice, alcohol, or soda) or did you fill up on bread? If so, that may have caused you to get stuffed before dinner. This will leave you with loads of empty calories but no real food or nutrients to keep you satisfied, and you will indeed get hunger pains by the time you get home. Next time, try to drink water with your meal and go for a healthier appetizer. In the meantime, if dinner truly didn't satisfy you, try to eat something light (low-fat yogurt, scrambled eggs or a nut butter sandwich).

WHAT IS MORE IMPORTANT—THE AMOUNT OF CALORIES OR THE TYPE OF CALORIES YOU CONSUME IN A DAY?

If two people were allowed 1,600 calories per day and one chose to eat fruits, vegetables, whole grains, and lean proteins while the other person ate foods full of refined sugar, fried meat, and fatty and processed snacks, would you consider these equal? Other than having the same amount of calories, it's hard to say they are similar in any other way.

That's why just counting calories won't always result in weight loss. You need to look at where they're coming from, in addition to how many you have. A good combination of calories from carbs, fats, and protein will help your body efficiently metabolize them. By sourcing your calories from foods high in vitamins, minerals, fiber, and other essential nutrients, your body will have the fuel it needs to get through the day and store only what is necessary. So forget about focusing on only the total number of calories and remember, it's quality and quantity. Think of it like you do your age: as Abe Lincoln said, "In the end, it's not the years in your life that count. It's the life in your years."

HOW MANY HOURS BEFORE BED SHOULD I STOP EATING IN ORDER TO AVOID A NIGHTMARE ON THE SCALE WHEN I WAKE UP?

It's not about how many hours before bed you stop eating, but rather the total amount (and quality) of calories consumed over the course of a day. Think of your credit card bill—it's not each receipt that makes you break out in a cold sweat, but rather the sum of all your purchases when you get your monthly statement. In both cases, it's a good idea to set a budget.

The reason most people tend to put on weight due to night eating is the types of foods they choose. Rarely do they reach for a bag of baby carrots or vegetables. Late-night snacking usually involves indulging in all sorts of things—chips, popcorn, chocolate, cookies. If you tend to graze at night, stick to lighter options and avoid anything fried, greasy, or full of fat, since these foods are harder to digest and won't sit well in your stomach. As you're about to lie down for (hopefully) eight hours, you'll also want to stay away from spicy foods, as they can irritate your stomach.

IS A FASTING DIET A GOOD WAY TO CUT CALORIES?

Your instinct may tell you that fasting is the best way to lose weight, but that's not the case. The only thing fasting does quickly is cause havoc. While you may see results at first, you can seriously interfere with your body's metabolism and you won't get the long-term weight loss you want.

Not only is fasting bad for your health, more often than not, it will cause you to fixate on food, which may have the opposite effect than you intended. You'll be much hungrier, and once you're "allowed" to eat again, you will likely overeat, which can lead to unnecessary and additional calories. It will also counteract what you did the day before. What counts is calories in and calories out on an overall basis—not just one day versus another. Additionally, by being gluttonous one day and malnourished the next, you are going to confuse your body. You may even start to feel sick by going from an empty stomach to a full stomach. This goes against the way your body prefers to be nourished and can do more harm than good.

The only thing a fasting diet will do is get you nowhere fast. Your body needs nutrients from food, and there are other healthier and less drastic ways to lose weight.

DESSERT IS MY FAVORITE PART OF THE DAY, BUT I DON'T WANT TO LOOK LIKE A CREAM PUFF. WHAT'S THE HEALTHIEST OPTION?

Generally speaking, it's okay to treat yourself every day. There is no reason to deprive yourself as long as you keep it to a small sampling or a few bites.

The healthiest options would be a bowl of fruit - frozen grapes, Greek yogurt with berries, or an apple with peanut butter. However, there are times when we know that won't cut it. On those nights, try to keep it to 150 calories, which is equivalent to two to three squares of dark chocolate, a few small cookies, or an individual chocolate pudding. You could also choose a few spoonful's of ice cream or sorbet, a baked apple, a popsicle, or even a small brownie. The key word here is or, not and. While eating out, pick a dessert that the whole table will enjoy. Ask for extra spoons or forks so everyone can share—forced portion control! As long as you keep the portion size small, a moment on the lips won't last a lifetime on the hips.

SOURCES
PART I - NUTRITION

1. Harvard Health

2. Whole Foods Market

3. Google

4. He FJ, MacGregor GA. A comprehensive review on salt and health and current experience of worldwide salt reduction programmes. J Hum Hypertens. 2009;23:363-84

5. nhlbi.nih.gov

6. mynutrition.wsu.edu

7. water.usgs.gov

8. vox.com

SOURCES
PART II - EXERCISE

1. heart.org
2. healthfinder.gov
3. cdc.gov
4. nihseniorhealth.gov
5. health.harvard.edu
6. nhlbi.nih.gov
7. mayoclinic.org
8. eatright.org
9. livestrong.com
10. nhs.uk
11. runnersworld.com
12. greatest.com
13. active.com
14. nerdfitness.com
15. bodybuilding.com
16. ideafit.com
17. fitnowtraining.com
18. betterhealth.vic.gov.au

SOURCES
PART III - WEIGHT LOSS

1. Harvard Health

2. psychologyofeating.com

7198 7356

6112 8923

(800) 908-9946

4506 T

Q z g = J G ? X